SEXUAL AND SPIRITUAL REAWAKENING

Fourth Book in the *LOVE ME, TOUCH ME, HEAL ME* **Series**

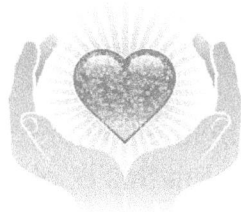

The Path to Physical, Emotional

Sexual and Spiritual Reawakening

Dr. Erica Goodstone

Publisher Data & Legal Information

Every attempt has been made by the author to provide acknowledgement of the sources used for the material in this book. If there has been an omission of any source, please contact the author at DrErica@DrEricaWellness.com

Disclaimer: No responsibility is assumed by the authors/publishers for any injury and/or damage and/or loss sustained in persons or property as a result of using this product; and/or for any liability, negligence or otherwise use or operation of any products, methods, instructions or ideas contained in the material herein.

The views and opinions expressed in this book and related materials are derived from the author's experience and research as a professor of health and physical education, yoga and meditation teacher, licensed mental health counselor, licensed professional counselor, licensed marriage and family therapist, board certified sex therapist, licensed massage and bodywork therapist, certified pain management practitioner, certified Integrative Medicine practitioner, certified Polarity Therapist, certified Rubenfeld Synergist, and involvement with numerous professional associations. She is not a licensed M.D. and does not diagnose or claim to cure any physical disease. She is also not a psychiatrist and does not claim to cure mental illness.

Any reader currently under the care or supervision of a psychiatrist, physician or other medical or behavioral health practitioner is urged to seek their professional advice before using or practicing any of the material or techniques contained herein.

Sexual and Spiritual Reawakening, **Book Four in the series, is dedicated to**

* Bryce Britton-Kranz, my friend, colleague and mentor in this powerful work that is so close to the human soul
* Dr. Alice Ladas, Grande Dame of research in female sexuality and body psychotherapy, who stepped out into a man's world as a pioneer and advocate, lighting the way for all the women that have and will follow
* Dr. William Masters and Virginia Johnson, who pioneered sex therapy, leading to the creation of a unique and gratifying profession
* Dr. Deryck Calderwood, my creative and courageous teacher, who taught me to stand on my own in the face of criticism and cynicism
* Dr. Mary Calderone, who reminded me that sexuality and love, are not and need not be, separate from love and the rest of our life
* American Association of Sex Educators, Counselors and Therapists, AASECT, for providing leadership, certification, and a place to call home among colleagues when I was a fledgling therapist
* Socicty for Scx Therapy and Research, SSTAR, for bringing together the leading authors, researchers, educators, psychotherapists, psychiatrists, and medical professionals to dialogue and explore sexual issues, concerns and treatment possibilities, through presentations and case studies
* Ilana Rubenfeld, my teacher and mentor, who encouraged me to forge my own way and create my own unique style of healing therapy, which I originally called *Sexual Reawakening*

ABOUT THE AUTHOR

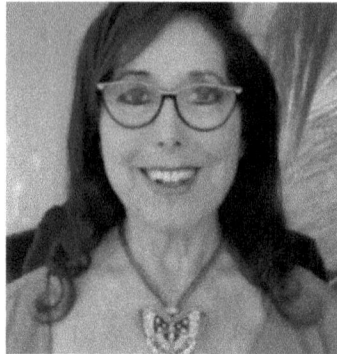

Erica Goodstone, Ph.D., has devoted her life's work to the discovery of love, healing and the creation of intimate, satisfying, fulfilling and joyful relationships. During over two decades, through her lectures, seminars and private counseling sessions, she has worked with thousands of men and women to create love and healing in their lives.

Having studied extensively from many different sources, Dr. Goodstone is a licensed mental health counselor, professional counselor, marriage and family therapist, massage and bodywork therapist. She is a diplomate and fellow for the American Association of Integrative Medicine and a diplomate for the American Academy of Pain Management. Dr. Goodstone is also a diplomate for the American Board of Sexology, a fellow for the American Academy of Clinical Sexologists, and a certified Sex Therapist for the American Association of Sexuality Educators and Therapists.

As a former professor of health and physical education at F.I.T./State University of New York, Dr. Goodstone spent 25 years studying and teaching about the body: physical fitness, health and wellness, stress management, sports psychology, team building and human sexuality. But she did not stop there.

Dr. Goodstone also spent many years studying a wide variety of healing body therapy modalities in including massage, shiatsu, polarity therapy, craniosacral therapy, Reiki, reflexology, Chinese medical theory, Japanese healing theories. Her studies led to the combination of touch with counseling through the gentle yet profound Rubenfeld Synergy Method. In fact, she was on the original steering committee and the board of directors for the first two terms of the U.S. Association for Body Psychotherapy. This was the first organization to bring together all the different originators and practitioners of somatic body psychotherapy methods and modalities.

But Dr. Goodstone's knowledge and background does not stop there. She has also fervently and passionately craved her own inner spiritual development and outer social awareness. Her seeking led her to spend many years studying yoga, first with the Sivananda Center in New York City and at the Sivananda Ashram in Paradise Island, Bahamas, where she met Swami Vishnu Devananda and listened to Ravi Shankar play the sitar. Later she spent years working with Guru Mayi, Swami Muktananda's disciple, receiving Darshan and personl counseling as needed.

Her studies included attending many consciousness raising seminars in the 1980's, including the EST seminars led by Werner Erhard, the Living Love Workshops led by Ken Keyes, Jr., author of *The Handbook to Higher Consciousness,* and DMA seminars about the creative process and structural thinking led by Robert Fritz.
She avidly studied the Rosicrucian manuals for many years, along with the Kaballah teachings of The Builders of the Adytum and the Course in Miracles. Her current focus has been exclusively upon the works of Joel Goldsmith, *The Infinite Way,* and Siddha Yoga Master Swami Muktananda.

Dr. Erica Goodstone has been a celebrated speaker at national and local professional and public events. Since her doctoral dissertation, which studied the effects of early mother-infant bonding upon later adult intimacy, she has continued to write extensively about creating love through the healing power of touch, intimacy, and the mind/body/spirit connection.

Dr. Goodstone's interviews and articles have appeared in *Who's Who of Medicine and Healthcare, CBS 4 TV, Blog Talk Radio Logical Soul Talk, Mademoiselle, Cosmopolitan , Marie Claire, Penthouse Forum, Journal of Sex and Marital therapy, Newsletters of the U.S. Association for Body Psychotherapy.* Dr. Goodstone has a very wide presence on the web. Her bio and blogs appear on numerous sites, e.g., Wordpress.com and Gather.com, as well as numerous ezines, most notably ezinearticles.com,

Dr. Goodstone's romantic novel, Love in the Blizzard of Life, as well as her books and Kindle books, are available at amazon.com. Her "Sexual Reawakening" chapter appears in the wonderfully organized book of Rubenfeld Synergy practitioners, *Healing Journeys: The Power of Rubenfeld Synergy, V. Mechner, Ed.* She has also written a section about touch therapies in the internationally acclaimed book, *The Continuum Complete International Encyclopedia of Sexuality*, R. J Noonan and R. Francoeur, Eds.

Dr. Goodstone can be reached at DrErica@DrEricaWellness.com

****

INTRODUCTION To The Series

Love Me, Touch Me, Heal Me: The Path to Physical, Emotional, Sexual and Spiritual Reawakening shows us what it takes to love, touch, and heal our own self. As we heal, we develop a renewed passion for life, a deep sense of being connected to something beyond our immediate life circumstances, and an increased desire for intimate loving. *Love Me, Touch Me, Heal Me* is meant to be a coming out party, coming out of hiding, bringing our total self into the light for examination, acceptance, and readiness to share our authentic self intimately with others.

Clients, colleagues and friends have often asked me to recommend a good book about love and relationships or about emotional intimacy and sexual communication. Others have requested information about ways to heal their body through natural methods, e.g., diet, exercise, body therapy, or even spirituality. And some have wondered what the best psychological approach might be to overcome fears, anxiety, anger, depression or relationship conflicts.

Answers to the above questions will be easily obtained as you read through this series of four ebooks. You will discover that you can find the answers to most of your problems, dilemmas, life issues and concerns through self-evaluation. As you complete the exercises, you will literally begin to heal your cellular memories, create new brain patterns and remove lifelong blocks to intimate joyful relating. You can turn to professionals for expert opinions, guidance, support and mentoring, but with this book you will begin to more fully trust your own inner knowing about what is truly best for your growth and healing.

FORMAT OF THIS BOOK

This **Book Series** is divided into four books consisting of three

chapters in each book as follows:

- Every chapter contains vital information, theories, concepts and suggestions gleaned from years of study, research, personal and professional experiences.

- Every chapter includes pertinent real-life stories, individual and partner written, verbal and contemplative exercises.

- Every chapter builds upon the previous one in the healing process.

- Every chapter is also complete unto itself.

- You may choose to read one entire book from start to finish and then begin a second book.

- You may choose to start with a specific chapter in any of the books.

- Resources, references, and keywords will appear at the end of each book.

This entire series of four books was originally intended to be one book. Written many years ago, this book has been hibernating in file boxes until now, a time when this world needs all the love we can muster. And this book teaches us how.

Love Me, Touch Me, Heal Me: The Path to Physical, Emotional, Sexual and Spiritual Reawakening belongs in the personal library of anyone who truly wants to heal from the past and create loving, touching and authentically intimate relationships. This is a guidebook, a reference book, and a comforting friend along the path to reawakening.

HOW TO USE THIS BOOK

This book is about your life, my life, and all of our lives. Read this book, follow the exercises, and watch miracles happen. *Love Me, Touch Me, Heal Me* is a life transforming healing process. For best results, you will need a few basic materials.

1. Writing Materials

a. **A journal, preferably a beautiful, special journal, but any 4" by 6" or 8" by 10" lined or unlined, notebook will do.** Choosing a journal or notebook that is special to you creates an experience of sensory stimulation every time you write in it! If you choose to write all the exercises in this book on pieces of paper, that's okay. But, if the outer appearance is appealing and soothing to your eyes, if the texture satisfies your sense of touch, if there's a fragrance of fresh cut paper or soft smooth leather that comforts you, the power of the words you write will be enhanced. Your brain will connect the sensual beauty of your journal with your written words and with your life. Your mind and body will begin to believe that you are serious about creating healing, love, spiritual connection, sexual aliveness, and joy in your life.

b.   **Pen, pencil, colored pencils or crayons.**

Brain research indicates that the mind absorbs information best when all the senses are involved. So get yourself a box of colored pencils, colored pens or crayons. You'll probably discover that you want some pastels, and maybe even paint and brushes before you're through. Colors and textures add additional dimensionality to your writing, increasing the possibility for your brain to record and store your hopes and dreams, uplifting words, goals, new beliefs, and appropriate affirmations. This allows your mind, at a later point in time, to easily refute your fears, frustrations and anxieties as they arise in your consciousness. Crayons and colored pencils may also stimulate your brain to create images, faces, doodles, and other self-expressions that reveal some important subconscious personal thought

Processes.

2. **_A quiet place, even a corner of a room, set aside to practice the exercises._**

    Energy accumulates in a space that you set aside and use specifically for one purpose. Creating a special place for your own inner work is a strong suggestion to your subconscious, (the part of your brain that allows your dreams to germinate into fruition), that you are serious about transforming your life.

3. **_Recording Materials_**

    Choose your own recording device.

    To do the exercises in this book, you can read and stop, read and stop, or you can record your own voice first. Then you will be able to go straight through the exercise without stopping. The goal is for you to comfort yourself and love yourself. Hearing your own voice is a powerful affirmation that you can create what you want and you are all you will ever truly need.

As you begin your journey along the path to love, take a moment to assess where you are right now in your life. The questions you are about to answer may seem simple but are actually quite profound. Observe your thoughts. Notice any automatic body responses you may have. You are more than your thoughts. You are more than your body. Allow your automatic responses to help you to discover who you truly are.

For all the exercises in this introduction and in the rest of this book, you have choices. You can read the exercise and then write in your journal. You can record the entire exercise with your own voice, close the book, close your eyes, and visualize freely. Or, you can listen to the pre-recorded audio tapes that accompany each chapter.

Who Are You?

Sit in a comfortable position.

Inhale slowly, very slowly, and deeply.

Exhale slower than your usual rate.

Take three slow, deep, easy, and quiet breaths.

Close your eyes and allow your body to relax.

Take three more slow, deep, easy, and quiet breaths.

Open your eyes only to read each question.

Immediately close your eyes and allow the answer to come to you.

Accept the answers that come. Do not edit or change the response

Listen to your mind's first answer, the most correct response at this moment.

> *Who am I?*
>
> *What are other people here for in my life?*
>
> *Why am I alive now?*
>
> *What do I believe about love?*
>
> *Who do I enjoy touching and for what purpose?*
>
> *What yearns to heal inside of me?*
>
> *What does sexual reawakening mean to me?*
>
> *What is the role of God, a higher power, or spirituality in my life?*

BOOK FOUR *SEXUAL AND SPIRITUAL REAWAKENING*

TABLE OF CONTENTS

SEXUAL AND

SPIRITUAL

REAWAKENING

BOOK FOUR

INTRODUCTION

We are all sexual beings. Sexuality teaches. Sexuality heals. Sometimes our sexuality hurts. When we allow our hearts to feel love and our bodies to feel pleasure, we are sexual. Being sexual is being alive. Feeling our sexual aliveness reawakens us to who we are. By allowing full sexual expression into our life, we cannot help but discover our spiritual nature.

We are all spiritual beings. Connecting to our spiritual nature and spiritual potential brings us an accepting appreciation of life. The path of discovering our spiritual connection can be difficult, painful and may reveal to us our deepest, darkest, most unloving personal attributes. Following a spiritual path also connects us to the highest values and the most life affirming self we can be.

Our life path is a spiritual path, the process of rediscovering our connection to all that is. No matter which direction we choose to take, all paths will eventually lead us home. Every spiritual teaching reminds us of that simple truth. If we resist knowing this truth and pursue a self-centered and purely material way of life, we may encounter more struggle, more difficulties, and more tests than necessary. But even if we do pursue a spiritual path, there are still obstacles and difficulties to be overcome. The difference is that knowing our spiritual essence provides emotional strength and calmness in the face of any stormy life issues, problems and concerns. *Sexual and Spiritual Reawakening* is a simple guide to help you live a more fulfilling, meaningful, and joyful existence.

****

SEXUAL AND SPIRITUAL REAWAKENING

"Use It Or Lose It."

Dr. William Masters and Virginia Johnson

"Love and Sex Go Together."

Dr. Mary Calderone

We are all spiritual and sexual beings. Sexuality teaches. Sexuality heals. Sometimes sexuality hurts. When we allow our heart to feel love and our body to feel pleasure, we are sexual. Being sexual is being alive. Being sexual reawakens us to who we are. As we reawaken, we realize that we are spiritual beings connected energetically to everyone and everything around us. In we explore what it means to be a spiritual and sexual being. We examine our current attitudes, beliefs and behaviors, our personal spiritual and sexual history, and how we can create and sustain our spirituality and sexual aliveness, even if we never attend another church service or never have a sexual partner again.

SEXUAL AND SPIRITUAL REAWAKENING

Becoming One

Take my hand

And join me

On the sacred path to love

Our hands entwined

And hearts engulfed

Our bodies throbbing

Sensing, glowing

Lost in sensual delight

Unaware of self

United

Connected

Belonging

Becoming

Knowing

We are One

Copyright ©   3/23/09 Erica Goodstone, Ph.D.

ORDINARY PEOPLE

ORDINARY

YET EXTRAORDINARY

SEX

SEXUAL AND SPIRITUAL REAWAKENING

CHAPTER 1

ORDINARY PEOPLE

ORDINARY YET EXTRAORDINARY SEX

ORDINARY PEOPLE

ORDINARY YET EXTRAORDINARY SEX

She smiles
He strokes her hair
She cries
He comforts her

He talks
She quietly listens
He screams
She calms his fear

They live together
In separate worlds
Sometimes sharing
Often, all alone

And then their bodies meet
The touch feels warm
Familiar
Safe

Though years of life
May mar their outer looks
Together they find love
Acceptance, joy

No special way
To look or be
Wrapped in arms of love
Their hearts are free

Copyright © 10/29/99 Erica Goodstone, Ph.D.

Sometimes In An Ordinary Place

Sometimes, when I am in an ordinary place in my everyday life – at the supermarket, buying a newspaper, walking down the street – I glance up at some complete stranger. It could be a man, some man, any man, and I wonder to myself,

Does this man enjoy sex, love women, or fear them both?

Does he know his own masculine beauty and manly strength?

Does he have a sexual problem or a compulsion?

Does he enjoy pleasuring his partner and does he teach his partner how to pleasure him?

I wonder for a while about this man of mind's moment and I walk on. Another man, another rmoment of thought….   Life's small capsules of universality revealed. All men are lovers. All men are sexual partners, at some time, with someone, if only in their dreams or with themselves.

At other times I notice a woman, some woman, any woman, and I wonder to myself,

Does this woman enjoy sex, love men, or fear them both?

Does she know her own feminine beauty and womanly strength?

Does she have a sexual problem or compulsion?

Does she enjoy pleasuring her partner and does she teach her partner how to pleasure her?

I wonder for a while about this woman of my mind's moment and I walk on. Another woman, another moment of thought…. Life's small capsules of universality revealed. All women are lovers. All women are sexual partners, at some time, with someone, if only in their dreams or with themselves.

On The Street

Next time you walk down a street, any street, pay attention randomly to different men and different women. Imagine what their sexual lives are like or may have been in the past. Imagine what their secrets or private fantasies might be . Observe couples. You may notice the most ordinary looking man or woman, someone you do not find particularly attractive, being hugged and cuddled by someone who obviously cares. You may also notice a very attractive, seemingly successful person being ignored or berated by an unloving partner.

Loving and being loved knows no boundaries. It is not based upon our physical appearance or our financial status. Yes, sometimes we are loved for some false physical or mental i8mage we have created or someone has created for us. But, as we open our hearts to another, pretense and illusion dissolve. Love endures when we are seen and accepted for who we really are.

The Average Man
And The Average Woman

The sexy media images have affected all of us. The ordinary man or woman dating another ordinary man or woman, may be unable to appreciate his or her very real partner. Many of us feel deprived, as if we are not getting our fair share of the love, excitement, money and youthful beauty that is out there for the taking.

Many of us also feel insecure about our ability to attract a desirable partner. Women spend thousands of dollars every year to alter hair color, reshape body proportions, and revitalize skin tone and texture. Breast implants, liposuction, face lifts and tummy tucks are quite popular surgeries for women. But even men have become increasingly concerned about physical appearance than ever before. Cosmetic surgeries to add inches to the penis while removing excess fat form the midsection have become big business in the medical profession

- **Ignore the media messages.**

- **Love the real people in your life.**

Just as we study for our degrees, work hard I our careers, and practice our favorite leisure activities, creating a magnificent relationship with open communication and exciting sex, requires single-minded focus on our chosen partner. With time, patience, concentration, devotion, acceptance and love, you can unleash the hidden passion in even the most reticent partner. You can find the gift of love with your very real and available partners.

Your Sexuality

At this point in your life, your sexuality may be flourishing, suppressed, unsatisfying, or just okay. You may be married or living with a partner in a monogamous, committed relationship. You may be sexually involved with many different partners or may have just lost a beloved partner through a breakup, betrayal, or even death. And perhaps you have never experienced a satisfying intimate relationship.

If you feel your current sex life is satisfying, then sexual reawakening may not be fore you. But if, like so many of us, your sex life has always been or has recently become less than fulfilling, you may decide you want more out of life.

Are you satisfied with your current sexuality, the way you look, the way you feel, and your ability to express yourself intimately with a partner? Is there something you would like to change, improve or experience, perhaps for the very first time?

As you begin the process of sexual reawakening, you gradually uncover and transform your life issues, fears, and intimacy avoidance strategies. According to the Dalai Lama (*The Art of Happiness*, 1998), happiness is the most important goal of life. No matter where you are right now, you truly have the God-given ability to create happiness in all areas of your life, including your most intimate sexuality.

Sex Doesn't Live Here Anymore

Given up on love and sex? Too much trouble…. Too unsettling…. Life is easier, alone, without a partner and without the hassles. If you've been feeling this way, you certainly are not alone. Many of us choose to remain single without a partner or maintain our own separate life within an emotionally unfulfilling marriage or live-in arrangement. We may feel unhappy, but we may also feel safe. Alone in our own world, we know who we are, we feel okay about ourselves, and we are able to go on living. Some of us fill our lives with work, activities, social events, family, friends, and intimate conversations. But we are often starving to be touched, held, and loved, with or without intimate sexuality.

When Viagra, the alleged miracle erection drug, was released in the Spring of 1998, the media revealed that over thirty million men were having erectile problems. What an astounding statistic! And those are the men who had discussed this problem with their medical doctors or therapists. What about men struggling with impotence and other sexual problems who have never told a doctor? What about all the women who suffer silently with their own sense of sexual inadequacy?

Many of us are uncomfortable in our own bodies, feeling overweight, in poor physical condition, or suffering from chronic physical and emotional ailments. When you are physically or emotionally uncomfortable or worried about some aspect of your life, your sexuality becomes less important than overcoming your very real problems. Anxiety and fear are often the antithesis of sexual potency.

Whether you are single, married, cohabiting, widowed, separated or divorced, you may at times feel anxious and uncertain about your sexual performance or you may sometimes worry about losing your sexual appeal. Frustrated that you cannot find a partner or angry at your current unresponsive and inept partner who does not satisfy your sexual needs, you may be living a life of quiet sexual desperation. You may long to hold on to something you once had, never quite had, or feel you are losing. You may not know where to turn or what to do.

Talking to your doctor about your intimacy concerns is not always helpful. Few physicians, and not very many psychotherapists, are trained to deal effectively with sexual issues. Regardless of the problem, you may be told, "Don't worry about it. At your age, that's normal." Many doctors assume that a man over 40 or 50 or 60 will naturally have a lower sexual drive, lose his erection sometimes and have decreasing pleasurable sensations. Some doctors actually advise women approaching menopause that vaginal pain is something they will just have to live with, that lessened sensation or numbness is normal, and that fewer and less pleasurable orgasms are to be expected.

Not true! There are men and women, who may have felt little sexual arousal when they were younger, that finally begin opening up to their sexuality in their mid-40's, 60's or even 80's. Many couples enjoy their best sexual experiences in their later years when they are no longer burdened by heavy financial, family and emotional responsibilities. In fact, women and men in nursing homes, who are not physically incapacitated, may enjoy sexual intimacy if the facility management is not too restrictive and they are able to find an available partner .

Your level of sexual enjoyment and satisfaction has very little to do with your age, physical attributes, or relationship situation. Regardless of how physically and emotionally intimate you are with another person, your sex life can be flourishing, exciting, a powerful stress reliever or it can become a major source of frustration and misery in your life.

It doesn't matter if you are married or living with a steady partner, engaged to be married, involved with many different partners simultaneously, recently ended a love relationship, lost a beloved partner through rejection or death, or have had a lifelong habit of pursuing non-intimate sex with or without a partner.

Take A Lesson From Mrs. Kalish

A few years ago I received a phone call from a childhood neighbor, an acquaintance of my mother, someone I had not seen for over 20 years. After we caught up on the news from the old neighborhood, she said, "By the way, I have a new boyfriend for the past three years. My previous relationship lasted about 10 years." In my mind I was calculating, "How old can she be?" My mother passed away a few years ago at the age of 76. Maybe Mrs. Kalish was younger. I figured by now she must be about 74 or 75. That's when the clinker hit me.

"I bet you're curious about my age", she said, as if she had read my mind. "I'm 89. and my boyfriend is 93. And I'm having the time of my life.

We see each other almost every day. He's a good man - and so much fun. We go to the theater and dancing. This weekend we're going to the beach. My life is pretty happy now. I'm lucky." Before saying goodbye, she asked me if I was lecturing somewhere, saying she would love to come.

Are you really "too old" at 25, 40, 55 or 70 to find love, romance and sexual intimacy? Is it true that "all the good ones are taken?" Do you believe you no longer have the energy for dating at your age? What I learned from Mrs. Kalish is that love and sexuality, romance, happiness and joy, is available to us throughout our lives.

What Do We Know About Sex?

Our sexuality is deeply connected to who we are. If we are having problems in this area of our lives, we may believe there is something wrong with us. Another, more positive and hopeful approach is to view sexual problems as messages about our lives. Our bodies often feel what our minds may refuse to acknowledge. Our bodies remind us to pay attention to ourselves, to listen to our own internal responses.

Researchers Masters and Johnson have claimed that our sexual organs are designed to function naturally, unless interfered with in some way.

During normal sleep, healthy males have an erection every 80-90 minutes and healthy females lubricate vaginally every 80-90 minutes. Medication, illness, injuries, surgeries, stress, relationship problems and other emotional upsets can and often do interfere with our normal sexual functioning, even during sleep.

It has been said that men think about sex every 6 to 8 seconds. If this is true, why do so many men nowadays have low sexual desire, inability to maintain an erection, and not so pleasurable feelings during ejaculation? If sex is a natural function, why are so many women lacking in desire and unable to have orgasms? And why are so many couples unable to maintain their desire over the years.

Sex has become a real conflict for many people in our society. Men and women are often angry with each other, angry at themselves, frustrated, and lacking desire. Men are expected to always be ready for sex, to "perform" upon request, to be sexually confident and to know exactly how to pleasure a woman. Women are expected to "be sexy" yet chaste, to show off their bodies, to be easily orgasmic, and to know exactly how to pleasure a man. Both are expected to have high sexual desire and be perpetually turned on, no matter what experiences they have had or not had, no matter what has transpired in their current relationship, no matter how they feel about their partner.

Sexual Response
Is A Barometer of What We Feel

Sexual response is often a barometer of what we feel. If a man dates a new woman, takes her home, feels turned on and then loses his erection, his first reaction usually is: "What's wrong with me?" Perhaps he should ask: "What's right with me?" What is my body telling me? What does she say or do that makes my body tighten up and not want to feel? What memories or fears are being aroused when I'm with her? Do I feel guilty, angry or upset about something? Do I feel safe and secure, manly and significant with this woman?

If a woman does not feel aroused by her lover, her usual response is: "What's wrong with me?" Perhaps she should ask: "What's right with me?" What is my body telling me? What does he say or do that makes my body tighten and not want to feel? What memories or fears are being aroused when I'm with him? Do I feel guilty, angry or upset about something? Do I feel safe and secure, womanly and significant with this man?

Men often complain that there aren't any good women out there. Upon closer observation they may desire a fantasy type woman, one who is totally unavailable. They may fear that women want something from them, so they purposely withhold their love and affection. Unable to get close to a woman, they may eventually feel like giving up, hoping that someday their sex drive and desire will go away.

Women often complain that there aren't any good men out there. They may say that men are domineering, selfish and inconsiderate or nice but not exciting. In looking for excitement, however, they often choose men with psychological problems, addictive or abusive behaviors. Unable to get close to a man, they may eventually they feel like giving up, hoping that someday their sex drive and desire will go away.

When relationships and other people seem difficult or impossible, we need to reevaluate our own lives. We can reawaken something inside of us that will allow us to connect with others in a new way. We can rekindle something in our current relationship or disconnect, grieve our loss, and seek a new, more fulfilling relationship with a more available partner.

Opposites Attract

Mantak Chia, the author of numerous books on The Taoist energetic theories of love and sex, believes: "The flattening of sexual desire between regular partners is due largely to depletion of polarity or sexual-electrical tension." He claims that sexual-electrical tension results from the polarity that exists when two people exhibit opposite and different traits and behaviors. In other words, sexual desire increases when there are differences and conflicts, and diminishes when two people feel too easily compatible, peaceful and calm.

Japanese healing arts describe the universal energy as a balance between two opposing forces, yin, feminine (receptive, cold, dark) and yang (masculine, active, hot, light). Hindus refer to these energies as the balance between Shiva and Shakti. A scientist might analyze the attraction as the meeting of positive and negative poles of a magnet. In magnets, opposites attract, like repels.

Modern psychology offers us the term "codependency" to describe the relationship between two people with opposite yet complementary needs. Neither feels whole without the qualities and behaviors of their codependent partner. In a codependent relationship, the strength of each partner is dependent upon the other person sacrificing a part of themselves, not developing to their fullest potential. But opposites can and do co-exist in full expression in the universe. The energy of shiva and shakti, yin and yang, positive and negative magnetic poles, flow easily back and forth, with a mutual respect for the right of each to exist and self-express.

Without the attraction of opposites, there would be little reason for man and woman to connect, to procreate, and continue the human species. Perhaps, there would also be less emotional pain. But we would be missing the joy, mystery, wonder and excitement that comes from relating to a person with qualities different from our own. How can we know pleasure when we have never known pain? How can a man truly know what it is to be a man without ever knowing a woman? How can a woman truly know what it is to be a woman without ever knowing a man? Deeply knowing an intimate partner involves accepting and honoring our differences, exploring our similarities, and communicating with each other.

Many of us find it difficult or impossible to be turned on by the "right" person, the one who appears to have everything we say we want. In fact, what tends to work best is sex with the "wrong" person, one who doesn't fit our personal relationship criteria. The one who instills passion in us is likely to be the person who does not behave the way we would like, who causes us to feel frustrated, confused, and even angry.

Freud and later researchers concluded that frustration and even hostility often leads to sexual attraction and desire. One explanation may be biological. The limbic system, a set of structures in the interior of the brain believed to be important for sexual behavior, lies very close to the centers of pleasure and aggression.

Close association and easy access, through steady dating, living together, or marriage, can easily dampen our desire. With a new lover, feeling naturally somewhat anxious, and uncertain about the future, we often feel more alert, attentive and turned on.

In this society, we tend to ignore the polarities, sometimes favoring one sex at the expense of the other. We may temporarily lessen the conflicts but will ultimately also lessen the desire, passion and love. Let's bring back the passion, understand and enjoy our differences.

Your Opposite Attractions

Have any of your partners, previous or current, had traits that seemed to be directly opposite of your own?

How did that affect your relationship?

Were you able to accept your differences?

Did one or both of you attempt to change/transform the other?

What happened to the quality of your life together?

Sexual Relating

When I tell people I'm a sex therapist, women often ask: "Why do men always want sex? I want to spend some time so I can get to know him first. Before answering, I usually reflect upon the many men who have asked me, "Why do women always want to get emotionally involved so soon? Why can't I meet a woman who doesn't always pressure me to make a commitment?"

Why do men always want sex? Why do women always want commitment? Let's set the record straight right here and now. To begin with, not all men pressure women to have sex. To many men, sexual intimacy is downright scary. Feeling clumsy, inadequate, unskilled or even dirty, some men totally avoid sexual contact. And many women are freely sexual with a man they desire, following their passion and lust, without love or need for commitment. In fact, a large number of women prefer the challenge of trying to win the heart of an unreliable and self-centered "bad body," someone they can rightfully blame for problems in the relationship, rather than being personally accountable to a steady, reliable partner. A large number of men are truly sensitive, romantic and loyal lovers, showing respect and concern for their partners, while some women are demanding and insensitive. Nowadays, with the threat of AIDS and other debilitating sexually transmitted diseases, both men and women often prefer to know their partners for awhile before becoming sexually involved.

According to sociobiologists, a "normal", "healthy", "unrepressed" male probably does want sex most of the time. Sociobiologists claim that, having evolved from lower animals, human instinctual behavior is not that unique. The survival of most species depends upon the male impregnating as many females as possible in order to carry on the species. In the human male, each ejaculation contains millions of sperm, but most die almost immediately upon entering the female vagina. Among those that survive, only one single sperm cell may survive the long journey up the vaginal canal and actually penetrate the barriers surrounding the female's egg. Just as the individual sperm cells compete with each other, adult males compete with other males to attain the prize, the most beautiful, most fit, and most impregnable woman.

Why is it not in women's best interest, biologically, to have sex with numerous men? According to sociobiologists, women have natural limitations. They are born with a finite number of eggs, 400,000-600,000. Each month from puberty to menopause, usually only one egg matures and is released from the ovary into the fallopian tube, available to become fertilized by one sperm cell from one male. Conception to birth requires approximately nine months of pregnancy, during which time the woman's activities are often naturally restricted. Engaging in sexual activity promiscuously increases a woman's chance of being infected with a sexually transmitted disease which may compromise her fertility later on. It is in the woman's best interest to choose her male partner wisely. For if he does not provide adequate support, she will bear full responsibility of caring for the physical and emotional survival of her children alone.

Why do men tend to want to have sex all the time? They have little to lose and everything to gain by spreading their seed with numerous partners. Why do women usually prefer to wait to get to know a man better? She has everything to lose reproductively.

What Do Men Say They Want?

Women often talk among themselves about what they "think" men want in a woman. Women may believe that men want them to look like a gorgeous model, behave like a properly mannered heiress, and be cool, aloof and disinterested. Yes, among the hundreds of men with whom I've spoken, a small number actually do have very high-line requirements for the eligible women in their lives. Most men say they are looking for something much more simple and attainable. Here's what some men say they want:

"I don't believe I should look for someone to marry. I think I should go out and have good times. When I enjoy being with someone so much that I don't want to be without that person, because we're happy together, then I might decide to get married." Arnie, salesman

"I want a woman who is feminine and soft, not afraid to let a man feel like a man. A man who has pressure and problems at work wants to come home to a woman who will soothe him, massage him and touch him tenderly. I love cuddling and hugging. I think it's a normal need." Roberto, corporate executive

"I might just remain single. I fly planes in my spare time. We have a whole group of guys that take trips to exotic places several times a year. We like adventure, scuba diving, meeting new people from all parts of the world. Some of the guys have gotten married and their wives don't let them come on these trips anymore. I would want my wife to understand my need for adventure and time alone with the guys." Gary, entrepeneur.

"I guess I never really learned to trust a woman, never really wanted to get too close. I'm a pilot, so I'm home for a few days, then off to Boston, Paris, Cairo, Brussels. I have to have a certain kind of understanding in my relationships. Having been independent for so long, I'm 44 years old, I now realize what's important: to get close and to share my inner thoughts with one special person. It's the only way the world can work." Roger, pilot.

"My mother took care of my sister and me since my father died when I was three. I have seen how hard she worked and how much she cared about us. I want a woman who is not afraid to work and to work hard, but I am very willing to share the load and support her. If she's stressed out and upset, I want to be there for her. But I also want her to support me when I need help or comfort or understanding. I want us to share our lives together." William, electrician.

Do these comments sound like men are only looking for stop dead good looks and hot sex?

Ask Men

Ask the men you know, at work, at school, at parties, at the gym, in your neighborhood, at the supermarket, anywhere and everywhere you go, what they want in a woman. Ask the single men what they are looking for. Ask the married men what makes them happy. Their answers might surprise you and actually relieve that insecure anxiety that you just can't measure up to some perfect ideal you've been imagining. Men and women need each other as companions to go through life.

What Do Women Say They Want?

Men often talk among themselves about what they "think" women want in a man. Many believe that women want them to be rich and powerful, handsome, built like a weight lifter, aggressive, and highly sexual. Yes, among the hundreds of women with whom I've spoken, a small number actually do have very high-line requirements for the eligible men in their lives. But the majority of women say they are looking for something much more simple and attainable. Here's what some women say they want:

"I want a man who is focused on me. I don't want to feel uncomfortable when we walk down the street and a pretty girl walks by. I guess I'm insecure, but I want to know he thinks I'm special and isn't that interested in other women." Jane, freelance writer

"I'm tired of these immature men. I want a man who can stand on his own too feet, pay his own bills, and stand up for himself. I don't like bossy, controlling men, but I also don't want to be able to push him around. I want to know I have met my match both socially and intellectually." Alice, corporate vice president

"Men often expect too much from me. I work hard and need the man in my life to be able to accept that. I want a man who lives a full life, with friends, activities, business, even travel. Our time together is special to me, but I need to devote a lot of time to my profession. If he's too needy, I want to run the other way, and fast!" Letitia, psychiatric nurse

"I want a man to be the father of my children. If he can afford it, I would like to be an old fashioned housewife. I'd be happy to cook, maybe get some help with the cleaning, and take care of the home and our children.

To me, family life is the most important thing. I come from a large family and always dreamed of having lots of children." Jane, administrative assistant

"My husband died a few years ago. Sometimes I feel very lonely. Yes, I enjoy my evenings out with my friends. But I get tired of being only with the ladies. I want to hold hands with a man and feel like a couple again. I really want a companion to share my later years with me." Sonia, retired teacher

Ask Women

Ask the women you know, at work, at school, at parties, at the gym, in your neighborhood, at the supermarket, anywhere and everywhere you go, what they want in a man. Ask the single women what they are looking for. Ask the married women what makes them happy.

Their answers might surprise you and actually relieve that insecure anxiety that you just can't measure up to some perfect ideal you've been imagining. Men and women need each other as companions to go through life. The average man or woman wants the best partner available to share life's ups and downs, to create a family together, to have a sense of belonging, being loved, accepted, connected and not alone.

Marriage And Divorce On The Internet

It was Saturday night. Searching through the mental health chat groups, I discovered "Marriage, Separation and Divorce". My curiosity peaked, I figured I would just check this out, read one or two, and log off. Hours later, I was still reading messages that had been posted over the years.

What a heartwarming experience! Men and women, different ages, nationalities, economic status, life stages, are talking freely, openly, uninhibitedly about their personal marital dilemmas, all presumably from their own homes. Fascinated, I read story after story about the dilemmas and confusions of married life - little or no sex, sexual dysfunctions, money problems, physical abuse, no communication, loss of desire or interest in the mate.

I was touched by the wise, compassionate responses others had given to the "unhappily married" pleas for help and understanding. Never before has there been so much help, comradery and free expression, without the shame, guilt and judgments we fear receiving from our families and friends when we feel most vulnerable.

Your Online Chat

In this exercise, your task is to go online and find out what sites are available to you. However, **if you have a problem, a compulsive need to seek out online sites, then please refrain from doing this exercise**. Instead, recall some of the sites you have visited before. For those of you who have not yet done so, find a chat room, preferably at no cost, with an ongoing discussion about relationships and sexuality. Read the dialogue that has accumulated over time. If you choose to, write in some of your own responses and reactions. Compare what people are saying to the way you currently feel or have felt in the past about your own relationships. If you want, write what you have discovered in your journal. The goal of this exercise is for you to discover what other people are saying and how they are handling situations that may be similar to your own.

Hot Sex On The Web

The internet provides us with a source of comfort, friendship and connection with people we could not meet in any other way. Communicating on the net, we can become anything we choose to be. A person who is generally indecisive, insecure, compulsive, self-serving or insecure in their ordinary life may present an entirely different image with a few carefully chosen words. TV has provided us with many real life scenarios to help us cope better with our own lives. On the web, anything and everything is available. Sensual and sexual fantasy and fulfillment are only a mouse click away. The distinction between reality and fantasy is often blurred. Our real life partners cannot hope to compete with these better than life fantasy relationships.

This is not natural sexuality and certainly not sexual reawakening.
Only humans pursue non-contact, non-touching means to satisfy their sexual desires. Although many of us prefer to share ourselves with our intimate partners, a growing number of people have been using the internet and other non-intimate sources (massage parlors, lap dancing, phone sex) to fulfill their sexual needs. Many men and women are partaking of these non-

intimate services, sometimes for a lot of money and often at an even greater emotional cost.

We have lost touch with what it means to be human, to connect with another whole human being. Somehow our parents and grandparents knew how to see and accept and love the whole person. As my mother gained weight and grew to a size 16, my father lovingly repeated, "There's more of her to love."

Nowadays, when our partner gains weight or in some other way is not as physically fit, mentally attuned, or financially stable as we expect them to be, we tend to lose our sexual desire. Turning away from the real person in our lives, we may turn to the media or look elsewhere for the unattainable ideal.

Our partner who has gained weight or whose career has hit a downward bump, may actually be at the highest point of their inner awareness. Not being accepted for who they are can lead to resentment, anger and erosion of trust and intimacy. In essence they may feel, "If you won't accept me the way I am, I am no longer willing to accept you the way you are."

It is often easier to avoid facing our own feelings through non-intimate, fantasy sexuality than to share our most intimate thoughts and fantasies with a real human being.

There appears to be very little support, in the media or even among our closest friends, for sharing sexual pleasure with our real-life partners. We need to learn how to become close to and love a real person, not in spite of their availability and ordinariness, but because of their availability and ordinariness!

Exploring Internet Sexuality

In this exercise, you are being asked to go exploring through the internet. However, if you have a problem, a need to compulsively go to online sites, then your task is to just recall, without actually logging in and checking any sites.

Look for or recall those explicitly sexual web sites you have either been seeking or avoiding.

Locate a Virtual Community, create your own unique Avatar, and go socializing there.

Examine what you find with a critical eye, without judgment.

Ask yourself very honestly,

Is this what sexuality is all about?

Does virtual sexuality bring me the joy, pleasure, connection and comfort I desire?

What are the benefits or dangers of explicit sexuality online?

What are the benefits or dangers of romantic encounters online?

Good Sex

As a clinical mental health counselor, marital therapist and sex therapist for several decades, I have observed hundreds of men and women as I listened to their stories and sometimes heart wrenching relationship woes. A good sexual relationship is certainly not a "given." Many of us don't place sex as a high priority. We may choose our partners for logical, rather than sensual or emotional reasons. "He's such a good man." "She's kind and nurturing." "He's so handy, he takes care of everything for me." "Sex with her is just okay, but she's a terrific cook and would make a wonderful mother." A good number of us choose a partner with whom we feel safe, someone with whom we may feel a close friendship but very little sexual desire. Many of us are afraid of our own sexual feelings.

Being with someone who does not arouse our sexual passion can give us the false impression that we are not very sexual, that we don't care about sex, need sex, or even like sex. But our bodies will only close down for so long. We may find ourselves dreaming about intimate sexual encounters with strangers and people we barely know. Some of us only become sexually aroused by people who are unavailable and do not appear to need us or love us. In our minds, we may connect love with weakness, vulnerability with inadequacy. We may reject our very real, caring partner in search of some elusive fantasy.

Most of us assume the other person should know how to treat us sexually or should immediately be exactly like or different from our previous lover. We forget how long it may have taken to "get it right" in the past. Or, perhaps, there is no previous lover and we expect this person to make up for all the relationships we never had. Many of us can't even begin to see the other person at first. All we really see is how this person is similar to or different from our past lovers, members of our family, or our closest friends.

We come to our relationships with memories of our past experiences, good and bad, joyful and painful. Although we may verbally express the need and desire for an intimate relationship, we may also have very real fears about getting close to anyone. The barriers to intimacy are often stronger than we realize.

Good Sex for You

Sit quietly, close your eyes, and imagine the most wonderful and perfect sexual experience for you. *Who are you involved with, if anyone? What activities are you participating in? How do you look, feel and express yourself?* Take an imaginary snapshot of your "Good Sex" situation. In the next chapter, we will be exploring all the possible factors that have affected you and may be interfering with your ability to create and have the sexual experiences your desire.

It's The Little Things That Count

What do you focus on in selecting a new lover or a lifetime mate? Many men and women seek a partner who we believe can provide financial security for us, pay our bills, supply us with recreational money, and buy us gifts. Others accept a partner who contributes little or no actual money but provides us with "something" in return for our paying the bills. For some, a dynamite sexual relationship or a very attractive partner that one is proud to be seen with, is enough. For others, a partner who builds and repairs things, a partner who cooks, cleans and takes care of details, is enough for us to choose to stay together.

Usually, some combination of the above, plus more, is what it takes to maintain a relationship. A popular song in the 1950's summed it up in the title: *Little Things Mean A Lot*. The lyrics included the following: *"...say I look nice when I'm not. Touch my hair as you pass my chair, Little Things Mean A Lot. Give me your arm as we cross the street. Call me at six on the dot .... Give me your hand when I've lost the way. Give me your shoulder to cry on. Whether the day is bright or gray, give me your heart to rely on."*

Each of us has those "little things" that mean more, or perhaps are equally as important to us, as money, power, good looks, or passionate sexual intimacy. Identify those "little things" that matter and choose a partner who naturally and easily provides them. Yes, we can train a reluctant partner to do some of those little things we like. But teaching and learning is a slow process, often takes a very long time, requires a great deal of patience, and sometimes results in very little change.

Look inside yourself. *Do you have the patience and perseverance required to teach and persuade your partner to provide those little things for you? Or would you rather switch than fight?* Know yourself and decide. One warning, however: Often, the partner who easily provides us with the little things, does not provide one or more of the "big" things. Conversely, a partner who provides the "big" things, such as money or passionate sex, may not easily provide the little things. The choice is always ours. Choose carefully. Our choice may remain with us for a lifetime!

The Little Things that Count for You

Think about your most passionate and exciting personal sexual experiences. Think about passionate scenes in movies, plays and other people's lives that truly moved you. Think about the types of seemingly unimportant slights, thoughtlessness, and forgetfulness that truly upset you.

In your journal or on a clean piece of paper write the heading, *"Little Things that Count."* Now, list as many of these little things that you can remember. Add to this list in the next few days and weeks as more little things that count occur to you.

Ordinary Can Be Extraordinary

Every relationship is a gift. Treat it that way. Let your partner feel like the beautiful Dulcinea or all-powerful Don Quixote in the play *The Man of La Mancha*. If you're currently in a relationship, imagine your partner saying the following words. **If you're not in a relationship, imagine the partner of your dreams saying these words.**

Just for today, be the man or woman of my dreams. Just for today, let me be the man or woman of your dreams. Just for today, give me your undivided love and attention. Just for today, let the miracle of love be ours.

Remember how special I am. I will remember how special you are. Remind me, over and over how much you love me. Look beneath my flaws and blemishes to my beautiful, perfect spirit within.

Treat me like a precious, innocent child, the one you love and adore, the one you shower with gifts. Protect me with your love from the harsh reality of the world. Listen to what I say I want and need. Whisper sweet, loving, kind words into my waiting ears. Tell me, without words, how much you care.

Love me for who I am and everything I want to be. Honor and respect my mind and body. Support me to reach for the highest in myself. Make love to me like you really mean it. Treat my body like a delicate, priceless work of art. Touch me tenderly and lovingly. Let me feel your magic at play.

Allow me to believe, just for now, that I am the only partner for you. Show you desire me. Hold me. Gaze into my eyes. Kiss my cheeks, my forehead, my eyelashes, my neck, my shoulders. Show me you desire me with your lips, your tongue, your voice, your heart. Massage away my fears, my aches and pains, and my heartfelt longing for love.

Gaze at me from a distance. Ignite my inner fire. Let passion between us build. Dance with me to the rhythm of sweet love. Please don't rush. We have time, lots of time - a lifetime, our lifetime. together.

TEN SIMPLE STEPS

TO

SEXUAL AND SPIRITUAL

REAWAKENING

SEXUAL AND SPIRITUAL REAWAKENING

CHAPTER 2

TEN SIMPLE STEPS TO SEXUAL AND SPIRITUAL REAWAKENING

Come With Me My Love

Come with me my love

Away to the countryside

Where we alone may know

The bliss and joy

And secret passion

Of every man and woman

That ever loved before

And those who may not

Yet have tasted

Life's sweet memories

Once known

Fulfills our sacred soul

With tender dreamy

Thoughtless peace

Tumultuous weary minds

Unwinding

Silent, quiet, still

Humble servants

Bowing their lowly heads

Before the almighty, omnipotent

Power

A single heart

Our heart -- beating as one

Awakened, alive and in love.

Copyright © 8/13/99 Erica Goodstone, Ph.D.

Your Unique Sexual Response Pattern

Each of us has a unique and individual sexual response pattern. This pattern mirrors and reflects the way we are living our lives. What appears to us to be a sexual problem is really a message from our subconscious, manifesting in our sexual response or lack of response.

When we are in our sexual prime and hormones are flooding our bodies, usually our teens to our early twenties, we may be able to easily override our body's subtle messages and willfully continue to "perform" sexually as our mind and ego choose. However, as we age and our hormones are more subdued, we reach a point when we can no longer forcefully override our bodily responses. Yes, we can take stimulants and injections to enhance our arousal, but the stimulating effect will eventually fade if we do not pay attention to the message our body is symbolically giving to us.

Your Body Is Stronger
Than Your Willpower

Even if we are able to override our unique sexual response pattern for a while, our body is stronger than our willpower. A poignant example is the case of a boy who, after a botched circumcision as an infant which left him with a mutilated penis, was reassigned as a female, given a female name, sex reassignment surgery and female hormones to encourage feminine development.

However, no matter how he was encouraged to dress and behave like a girl, his bodily response did not concur. He preferred to urinate standing up facing the toilet. He hated wearing dresses and walking the way he was taught a girl is supposed to walk. Teased mercilessly by his classmates in school for being weird and after spending years on the psychiatrist's couch to accept himself as a girl, when he was finally told the truth about his genetic maleness he was relieved. He knew than that he was not weird. He knew that he was in fact, male, with male traits, male drive, and male desire for females. His body had told him all his life what nobody else had been willing to say -- that he was a male being forced to live as a female. The gender reassignment did not work. Finally, after much reconstruction surgery and two suicide attempts, he emerged as a male and eventually found a woman to marry. (Colapinto, 2000)

Although this is an extreme example, many of us have likewise been attempting to override or suppress our unique sexual response in favor of some image we are attempting to portray. Attempting to hide our sensitive and caring nature, we may feign cool aloof standoffishness. Fearing closeness and intimacy, we may pretend to offer our partners emotional safety as we become increasingly anxious and uncomfortable. Desiring intimacy with a lifetime mate, we may pretend to enjoy one-night stands and non-committed sexual encounters. The list goes on. Our bodies may be quietly and sometimes not so quietly screaming for our attention.

We can continue the pretense for awhile, until our bodily responses finally begin to override our willpower and we are faced with a sexual problem. Without an obvious sexual problem, we might would go on indefinitely behaving in ways that are dramatically opposed to having what we want and are ultimately not satisfying to us. Our sexual problem may be the very catalyst that forces us to stop and examine, not only our sexuality, but the way we are living our lives and relating to others.

As we explore our sexuality, we have the opportunity for change and healing in all areas of our lives. We begin to pay attention to our bodies, what our bodies are telling us to do or stop doing. We listen to our minds, clarifying what we truly need and want. Feeling our emotions, we discover what is true for us. Paying attention to our senses, we feel more connected to the world and all it has to offer in this life.

Your Sexuality
Is Not Separate From Your Life

We discover that our sexuality is not separate from the rest of our lives and that our sexuality truly expresses who we are. As we begin to express who we are, life becomes a joyful experience, moment to moment. We feel love and compassion for ourselves and for everyone and everything around us. No longer feeling separate and alone, the world becomes a safe and pleasant place to be. Regardless of our age or physical condition, people are naturally drawn to our warm smile and pleasing demeanor. Love is all around us, everywhere we turn. Sexual Reawakening is the process that brings us back to ourselves, allowing us to open our hearts, give love to and receive love from our chosen partners.

Ten Simple Steps To

Sexual And Spiritual Reawakening

The following exercises will assist you to reawaken your sexuality, no matter where you are in your life at this very moment. If at all possible, please set aside a block of uninterrupted time before you begin. You can always do these exercises on different days, but the effect will be most powerful if you complete the entire process in one session. Have your journal or some plain white paper and a pen or pencil ready before you begin.

Factors That Have

Influenced Your Sexuality

You are about to review your own sexual history. This exercise may stir up feelings and memories you didn't even know you had. Have tissues nearby if you begin to cry. Have a pillow nearby to punch if you feel angry. In your journal or on a sheet of paper, write your answers to the questions. After completing each section, close your eyes and reflect upon that aspect of your sexual history.

The first, and probably most significant step along the path toward sexual reawakening, is to examine your current life, the way it is right now, not the way you wish it was, not the way you hope it will become, but the way it truly is right now. For some of us this is the most difficult step. If your style is to make excuses, blame others for your problems or deny that you have any problems at all, this first step may be hard for you to comprehend. However, with persistence and the willingness on your part to tell the truth, the whole truth, and nothing but the truth -- at least to yourself at first -- you may be surprised to discover how quickly your life begins to change.

STEP 1

Where Are You Right Now?

Your Current Relationship Status

And Your Sexual Lifestyle

Close your eyes. Take a few slow, deep, easy, and quiet breaths. As you inhale, allow your breath to fill your body cells and relax your muscles. As you exhale, allow the tensions of your body and the concerns of your mind to dissolve.

Your Current Lifestyle

What is your current living situation: married, separated, divorced, widowed, single, living with an intimate partner, living with your parents or other relatives, living in a room in your parent's home with a private entrance, living with a non-intimate roommate, living alone?

Are you financially independent, sharing expenses, or relying on someone else's income to support you?

Where do you live (city, suburbs, country)?

What are your current home and work environments like for you?

What is your current financial situation?

What is your daily activity and stress level?

What is your typical daily diet?

How much and what kind of exercise do you regularly do?

What types of drugs (prescription or recreational), vitamins or herbs do you regularly take and how have these affected you?

Do you have any unhealthy or compulsive habits: smoking cigarettes, drinking alcohol, overeating, dieting, overspending, gambling, sexual compulsions?

How have the above factors affected your life and your sexuality?

Have any aspects of your lifestyle changed? How? When? What caused the change? How does your current lifestyle affect your life and your sexuality?

Close your eyes and reflect upon your responses.

Your Gender Identity and Gender Roles

Are you satisfied with being male or female?

Do you ever wish you could be the other sex?

What do you believe males should do or be?

What do you believe females should do or be?

Do you fit your own idea of the way men or women should be and what they should do?

Do you fit what you believe is the way men or women should be in this society?

Has your satisfaction with being male or female changed? How? When? What caused the change?

Have your beliefs about male or female roles and behaviors changed? How? When? What caused the change?

How have your satisfaction with your gender and gender roles affected your life and your sexuality?

Close your eyes and reflect upon your responses.

Your Health: Physical, Emotional, Sexual And Spiritual

Think about any illnesses, operations, injuries, aches and pains, or other physical problems you are currently having or have had in the distant past or in the recent past.

Has your physical health changed? How? When? What caused the change?

How has your physical health affected your life and your sexuality?

Have you had any emotional upsets, traumas, or problems causing you distress, causing you to seek help or to take medication in the past? Recently? In the past?

Has your emotional health changed? How? When? What caused the change?

How has your emotional health affected your life and your sexuality?

Close your eyes and reflect upon your responses.

Your Age, Physical Appearance,

and Body Image

How old are you?

How do you feel about being your current age?

Are you comfortable or uncomfortable with your body as it is?

Has your physical appearance and comfort with your body image changed?

How? When? What caused the change?

How has the physical appearance of your body and your body image

affected your life, your sexuality and your spirituality?

What effect does your current age have upon your life and your sexuality?

Close your eyes and reflect upon your responses.

Your Partner Availability

How easy or difficult is it for you to find or connect with an available sexual

partner?

Has your partner availability changed? How? When? What caused the

change?

How has your partner availability or lack of availability affected your sexuality?

Close your eyes and reflect upon your responses.

Step Two

Where Did You Come From Originally?

Your Conception, Birth

And Earliest Years

The second step is to review your origins: your birth, early parenting, and how your earliest beginnings have affected your current life. For some of us, this second step is even more difficult that Step 1. However, if you've already practiced being totally honest with yourself, you may find your answers flowing easily. As you examine your origins, notice any judgements you may have, good and bad, about yourself, your parents or other caretakers, the way life has been for you, the way you believe life should be, what you feel you deserve or don't deserve, and the way life is.

You are about to go on an imaginary journey back to the moment of your own conception. Allow your mind to participate fully. Do not censor any thoughts that arise.

Allow your imagination to run free, recalling times you can only know intuitively.

Imagine that special date, 20, 30, 40, 50, 60, 70, or 80+ years ago, the moment when your mother and father performed the sexual act that created you.

Your Conception

How do you imagine your parents felt about each other before, during and after the moment when you were conceived?

Were either of your parents experiencing stress, physical or mental illness, under the influence of alcohol or drugs (prescription or recreational) while you were being conceived?

Close your eyes and reflect upon your responses.

Your Mother's Pregnancy Carrying You

How did your mother describe her pregnancy when she was carrying you?

Were there any complications?

How did she say she felt physically and emotionally?

How did she describe her sleep, exercise and rest?

Were your parents thrilled, conflicted or disturbed about your impending birth?

Did either of your parents want you to be the other sex?

Did your parents lose any children before you were born?

What effect did your mother's pregnancy have upon your life and your sexuality?

Close your eyes and reflect upon your responses.

Your Mother's Labor and Birthing of You

How did your mother describe her experience of labor when she was giving birth to you? How long did it last?

Was your father present in the delivery room and did he participate?

Who else was present in the delivery room?

Did you willingly and easily emerge or was there some dfifficulty?

Were you in a twisted or breech birth position?

Was the umbilical cord tangled around your neck?

Did you resist being born and find yourself pulled out with forceps?

Were you born through your mother's vaginal canal or cut out of her abdominal cavity by a caesarian section?

Were you born prematurely and were you placed in an incubator?

Was anything physically wrong with you when you were born?

What effect did your birthing process have upon your life and your sexuality?

Close your eyes and reflect upon your responses.

After Your Birth

How was your mother's physical and emotional health after your birth?

Were you breastfed and until what age?

Were you held and nurtured and by whom?

Did you sleep in the same bed or room with one or both parents or caretakers?

Were you left alone, neglected, or abused for any period of time?

What effect did your early infancy have upon your life and your sexuality?

Close your eyes and reflect upon your responses.

Step 3

What Happened Along the Way?

Your Sexual and Relationship History

Your Sexual Education

How was sexuality talked about and treated in your family of origin?

Who did you live with in your earliest years: mother, father, both parents,

relatives, adoptive parents, foster parents, siblings, or someone else?

Were your parents or early caretakers physically affectionate toward each

other.

Were your parents or early caretakers physically affectionate toward you?

Did you ever observe your parents or someone else in the sex act? How did

you respond?

Where and from whom did you learn about sexuality? At what ages?

Has your sexual education changed? How? When? What caused the change?

How has your sexual education affected your life and your sexuality?

Close your eyes and reflect upon your responses.

Your Earliest Sexual Relationships

Recall and describe your earliest sexual experiences, as an infant, young child, adolescent and teenager, as much as your memory will allow. For each stage of life, answer these same questions:

With whom were you involved? What happened? Who initiated?

Did you want to be involved or were you pressured, seduced, coerced or forced into submission against your will?

What emotions did you feel and were your feelings reciprocated by the other person?

How were you treated and how did you treat others?

What effect did those early experiences have upon your current sexuality?

Close your eyes and reflect upon your responses.

Your Adult Sexual Relationships

Recall and describe your most significant sexual relationships during each decade of your adult life (twenties, thirties, forties, fifties ...eighties....)

Describe your sexuality, how you felt about your body, your appearance, and your overall feeling about life.

Recall your hopes and dreams for your future.

Who loved and nurtured you and who neglected, abandoned or abused you?

Who did you love and nurture and who did you neglect, abandon or abuse?

Did your sexuality change? When? How? What caused the change?

How have your sexual relationships as an adult affected your life and your sexuality?

Close your eyes and reflect upon your responses.

The Significance of Your Sexual History

What events, situations, and people are significant in your sexual history?

How has your sexual history affected your life and your sexuality?

How has your sexual history, or what you know about it changed? Why?

Close your eyes and reflect upon your responses.

Step Four

Your Sexual Identity

And Partner Preferences

The Kinsey Heterosexual/Homosexual

Continuum

Many of us are confused about our sexual identity or sexual partner or object preferences. The Kinsey Continuum has been a useful source to help define for ourselves where they fit. In massive sexual surveys of the 1940's and 1950's, Alfred Kinsey and his colleagues discovered that most people exhibited degrees of homosexuality and heterosexuality, with bisexuality representing a midpoint. They created a seven-point heterosexual-homosexual continuum. People fit on the continuum according to two criteria: homosexual or heterosexual behavior and attraction to same sex or opposite sex. People in category "0," exclusively heterosexual, claimed no attraction, desire, or sexual activity, ever, with the same sex. People in category "6," exclusively homosexual, claimed no attraction, desire, or sexual activity, ever, with the opposite sex.

In Kinsey's studies, about 4 percent of men and 1-3 percent of women were categorized as exclusively homosexual, "6". A larger percentage were considered predominantly homosexual, "4" or "5", or predominantly heterosexual, "1" or "2". The largest percentage of people were classified as exclusively heterosexual, 50 - 92%. Thirty-seven percent of men and 13 percent of women claimed to have reached orgasm through homosexual activity at some time after puberty.

A 1970 nationwide survey conducted by the Kinsey Institute, a 1988 survey, and a 1993 Louis Harris poll, had results similar to the earlier Kinsey studies. Studies indicate that a large number of men and a smaller but still significant number of women have engaged in homosexual experience during their lives, and a very small percentage, 1-4%, within the last year to five years.

Where Do You Fit on the Kinsey Heterosexual/Homosexual Continuum?

Look at the Kinsey Heterosexual/Homosexual Continuum below. Circle the number that most accurately describes your experiences throughout your life.

0...... exclusively heterosexual, having had no homosexual experiences at any time in your life

1......almost exclusively heterosexual with one or more homosexual experiences

2......mostly heterosexual with some homosexual experiences

3......bisexual, indicating you have had sexual experiences with the same or opposite sex to about the same degree

4......mostly homosexual with some heterosexual experiences

5......almost exclusively homosexual with one or more heterosexual experiences

6......exclusively homosexual, having had no heteresexual experiences at any time in your life

THE KINSEY CONTINUUM

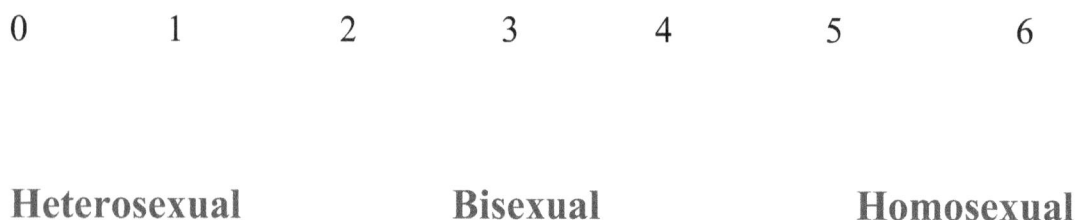

0	1	2	3	4	5	6

Heterosexual   **Bisexual**   **Homosexual**

(*Human Sexuality in a World of Diversity*, 1995)

Your Sexual Identity

and Partner Preferences

Where do you fit on the Kinsey Continuum?

Do you define yourself as heterosexual, bisexual, homosexual?

How do you feel about your sexual identity?

Have your sexual identity and partner preferences changed? How? When?

Why?

How have your sexual identity and partner preferences affected your life and

your sexuality?

Close your eyes and reflect upon your responses.

Step Five

Why Do You Want Sex?

What Do You Hope to Gain, Become or Experience?

Each of us has different reasons for choosing to have sexual relations with another person. At different times in our lives, we may have sex to feel pleasurable sensations, to play like children, to relieve tension, to alleviate pain, to avoid facing our problems, to feel comforted and touched, to express our emotions, to create a family, to explore our spirituality, or to discover our own true nature,.

Why Do You Want to Have Sex?

What is your reason for having sex or for currently not having sex?

What do you hope to learn, give, receive, become, or have through sexual contact?

What do you desire, fantasize and dream about?

How do you feel about having children or becoming a parent?

Do you want to have children with your current partner or with someone else?

How is sex better than touching, hugging, giving or receiving a massage?

Is there any other way for you to achieve the same sensations, feelings and goals?

How has your reason for wanting sex affected your life and your sexuality?

Close your eyes and reflect upon your responses.

Importance Of Sexuality In Your Life

How important is sexuality in your life?

Has the importance of sexuality in your life changed? How? When?

What caused the change?

How has the importance you have placed on sexuality affected your life and your sexuality?

Have you ever been celibate? For how long?

What effect did being celibate have, if any, upon your life and your sexuality?

Close your eyes and reflect upon your responses.

Your Current Sexuality

Are you currently being sexual with a partner: your spouse, live-in partner, casual date, steady partner, person other than your live-in partner, other?

How does your body feel before, during and after sexual relations with your current partner?

Are you currently celibate? For how long? For what reason?

How often do you stimulate yourself sexually and in what preferred ways?

Do you reach orgasm easily or with difficulty?

How do you feel before, during and after you stimulate yourself?

How does your current sexuality compare to each decade of your previous life?

What has remained the same? What has changed? When and how did it change?

When were you most happy, most fulfilled?

When were you least happy, least fulfilled?

What have you done in the past to improve your condition?

What are you doing now to improve your condition?

How is your current sexuality affecting your life?

Close your eyes and reflect upon your responses.

Your Sexual Function and Dysfunction

Are you satisfied or upset with your sexual functioning at this point in your life?

Are you currently experiencing any sexual problems?

* Desire problems

* Arousal problems

* Orgasmic problems

Have your problems been recent or lifelong?

Have these problems happened only in certain situations or in most circumstances?

Has your sexual functioning changed? How? When? What caused the change?

How have your sexual dysfunctions, if any, affected your life and your sexuality?

Close your eyes and reflect upon your responses.

So You Think You Have a Sexual Problem

When our bodies do not respond the way we think they "should," we are receiving a powerful message. Maybe we have been trying to force our bodies to do something we don't really want to do. Our brain sends the message to our pituitary, the master gland, signaling our ovaries or testes and other glands to secrete the hormones needed for us to become aroused. If our brain fails to send the proper signals, our glands will not secrete the needed hormones. We will either not become aroused, lose our arousal, or be unable to experience the pleasurable release of orgasm. We cannot ignore our body's messages and function with precision. We are not mere physical machines. We have a mind, emotions, five basic senses, a neuromuscular system, an autonomic nervous system, organs, tissues and glands -- and all of them affect each other.

Just as we cannot turn on a car ignition with the wrong key, insufficient gas or oil, a cracked starter, or worn spark plugs, we cannot "turn on" our sexual apparatus without the proper human fuel. That proper fuel is unique to each one of us and often different for the same person at different times. If we don't know what thoughts, feelings, visual images, words and sounds, physical sensations and moral principles ignite our private parts, then we may interpret our body's message as a sign that we have a problem, are not performing well, and are somehow inadequate.

Perhaps that "problem" that won't go away is merely our body's way of saying: "Pay attention to me."

Your Ideal Sexual Life

Close your eyes and imagine your sexual life being exactly the way you want it to be.

Where are you? Who is with you? What are you doing? How are you feeling?

Close your eyes and reflect upon your responses.

Step 6

What Is Your Sexual Style?

Sexual Pleasure, Variety

and Risk Taking Behavior

Many of us assume our friends have the same sexual desires and preferences that we have. Many of us believe that we can generalize and say that "men like...." and "women want...." Yet every one of us is a totally unique individual with our own fingerprint and specific DNA code. We have our own preferences and style in everything we do, from the way we eat, dress, work, play and talk to the types of friends and lovers we choose. Each of us has our own unique sexual style, needs, desires, interests and preferences. Why not allow our unique sexuality to emerge?

Through our intimate connections with others, we can resolve long held conflicts about our deepest sexual selves. Keeping our true sexual desires hidden from fear of being rejected, embarrassed or abandoned, we may be hurting ourselves or hurting someone else.

Sharing our sexuality in all its fullness offers our partners the opportunity to expand their own sexual expression.

Your Sexual Desire Level

What do you believe is your level of sexual desire: hyperactive (overactive), hypoactive (underactive), or moderate?

Has your desire level changed? How? When? What caused the change?

How has your sexual desire level affected your life and your sexuality?

Close your eyes and reflect upon your responses.

Your Sexual Arousal Style

How do you become aroused?

What type of stimulation or techniques do you require?

How long does it take?

Has your sexual arousal style changed? How? When? What caused the change?

How has your sexual arousal style affected your life and your sexuality?

Close your eyes and reflect upon your responses.

Your Sexual Orgasmic Style

How easily do you orgasm and how long does it take?

Do you have difficulty attaining orgasm?

Are you able to control the timing of your orgasm?

Does it take longer than you would like for you to have an orgasm? Why?

Does your orgasm happen sooner than you would like? Why?

Are your orgasms satisfying?

Has your orgasmic style or level of sensation changed? How? When?

What caused the change?

How has your orgasmic style affected your life and your sexuality?

Close your eyes and reflect upon your responses.

Your Sexual Resolution Style

How do you feel and behave after you have had an orgasm?

Are you affectionate, cold, indifferent, bored, restless, feeling guilty and ashamed?

Do you fall asleep, get out of bed, leave?

How do you feel waking up in the morning next to your partner?

Has your sexual resolution style changed? How? When?

What caused the change?

How has your sexual resolution style affected your life and your sexuality?

Close your eyes and reflect upon your responses.

Your Preferred
Sources of Sexual Stimulation

What is your preferred source of stimulation: visual images, auditory messages, kinesthetic, touch sensations?

Do you prefer to be the *recipient, victim, aggressor, perpetrator, or mutual partner?*

Which visual images, auditory messages, or kinesthetic sensations do you prefer: live person, intimate partner, strangers in the street, topless bars, call girls, prostitutes, massage parlors, videos, movies, internet sites, chat rooms, phone sex, magazines, photographs, self-pleasuring, other?

Have your preferred sources of stimulation change? How? When? Why?

How have your visual, auditory and kinesthetic preferences affected your sexuality and your life?

Close your eyes and reflect upon your responses.

Your Preferred Sexual Locations

At home: on a couch, in a bath or shower, in another room - explain, on a terrace, porch or outdoor area, hotel or motel room, automobile, public place with the danger of being caught, on a beach, in a hot tub, other

Which of the above sexual locations do you prefer? Which do you engage in frequently? Which have you seldom or never experienced?

In which locations have you been forced to have sex against your will?

In which locations would you like to have sex?

In which locations are you afraid to have sex?

Have your sexual location preferences changed? How? When?

What caused the change?

How have your sexual location preferences affected your life and your sexuality?

Close your eyes and reflect upon your responses.

Your Sexual Activity Preferences

Kissing on the lips, French or deep tongue kissing, sexual intercourse, cunnilingus, fellatio, anal Intercourse, analingus, fisting, sado-masochism, bondage, toys, role play, self-pleasuring alone, self-pleasuring with a partner present, ménage-a-trois, group sex, other

Which of the above sexual activities do you prefer?

Which do you engage in frequently?

Which activities have you seldom or never experienced?

Which activities have you been forced to do against your will?

Which sexual activities would you like to do?

Which sexual activities are you afraid to do?

Which sexual activities do you find disgusting or revolting?

Have your sexual activity preferences changed? How? When?

What caused the change?

How have your sexual activity preferences affected your life and your sexuality?

Close your eyes and reflect upon your responses.

Your Preferred Sexual Positions

Missionary Position -- man on top, woman on top, doggie style, spoon style -- woman's back to man, sideways -- facing each other, other specific positions, experiment with different positions

Which of the above sexual positions do you prefer?

Which sexual positions do you engage in frequently?

Which sexual positions have you seldom or never experienced?

Which sexual positions have you been forced to do against your will?

Which sexual positions would you like to do?

Which sexual positions are you afraid to do?

Have your preferred sexual positions changed? How? When? What caused the change? How have your preferred sexual positions affected your life and your sexuality?

Close your eyes and reflect upon your responses.

Your Sexual Performance Style

What is your sexual performance style: aggressive, passive, combination?

Is your sexual style narrowly focused and repetitive or multi-faceted and changing?

Is your style quick and fast or long and slow?

Has your sexual performance style changed? How? When? What caused the change? How has your sexual performance style affected your sexuality and your life?

Close your eyes and reflect upon your responses.

Your Sexual Pleasuring Style

Do you prefer pleasuring your partner?

Do you prefer being pleasured by your partner?

Do you prefer mutual giving and receiving of pleasure?

How has your preferred interaction style affected your sexuality, your life?

Has your sexual pleasuring style changed? How? When? Why?

Close your eyes and reflect upon your responses?

Your Sexual Communication Style

How easily do you communicate your needs to your partner?

How easily can your partner communicate his or her needs to you?

Has your sexual communication style changed? How? When? What caused the change? How has your sexual communication style affected your sexuality and your life?

Close your eyes and reflect upon your responses.

Your Sexual Commitment Style

Are you monogamous, choosing to stay with one partner for life?

Are you a serial monogamist, choosing to stay with one partner at a time, until the relationship ends?

Are you promiscuous, preferring to play the field sexually, with many different partners?

Has your sexual commitment style changed? How? When? Why?

How has your sexual commitment style affected your sexuality and your life?

Close your eyes and reflect upon your responses.

Step 7

What's Blocking Or Stopping You From Creating Joyful Intimate Sexual Relationships?

Sex Does Not Begin In The Bedroom

A man and woman enter the bedroom, tear off their clothes and jump into bed.

A married couple undress into their pajamas and meet each other under the covers.

Two people get into bed, turn their backs to each other, and turn out the light.

What happens next in bed is often the culmination of hours, days, weeks, months, even years, of courtship, loving interactions, or hostile exchanges, indifference, frustration, or even boredom. Sex does not begin in the bedroom. It starts with the way we look, act and interact with each other and by what we feel inside - all day long.

What interferes with our personal enjoyment of our own sexuality depends upon our unique experiences, our bodily and emotional memories of those events, and our current beliefs about love, sexuality and intimate relating. Our own personal programming determines our sexual responses. When we feel threatened by closeness, even the most gentle and tender touch by a loving partner may be perceived by us as pressure, demand, aggression, even violence. If we have been programmed to always please others, if we feel in any way inferior to our own idea of the way we should be, our sexual responsiveness may suffer. If we believe we are sexually inadequate in some way, we may fear that we will have to change. Change is always frightening because it involves the unknown.

The first step in reawakening our sexuality is to discover what is currently blocking or interfering with our ability to feel and enjoy pleasure. Some of us can only allow our sexual feelings to emerge when we are in the privacy of our own home, alone by ourselves. Some of us avoid physical contact even with our own body.

How Do You Look and Feel?

Stand in front of a mirror and observe yourself (with or without clothing).

Observe the way you are standing? Are you standing tall and proud, slouching, forcefully holding your body erect in a state of tension, or comfortably relaxed in your own presence?

Observe your breathing? Is it full and rhythmical or shallow and even held?

Observe your facial features, the quality of your skin, the expression on your face?

Are you looking your best or do you appear to be tired, older than your years, stressed out or relaxed and content?

Observe the rest of your body?

Are you satisfied with your physical appearance, your weight, your shape, your fitness level, your muscle tone?

Now go internally.

Are you satisfied with your personality and the way you present yourself to the world?

Are you satisfied with your life right now or is there something that you want to change?

What have your emotions been telling you about the way you are living your life?

Are you satisfied with your education, work, career, and finances or is there something you would like to change?

Are you satisfied with your family, your home life, and the quality of your intimate and non-intimate relationships?

Are you satisfied with the amount and quality of touching, loving, and sexual expressiveness in your personal life and most intimate relationships?

Taking a long, honest look at ourselves, our current lives, and what we truly desire, can be difficult, but well worth the time and effort. If we want a passionate sexual relationship, sometimes we need to change behaviors that are keeping people away. We may have to give more than we thought was necessary or not as much as we naturally give. We may have to ask ourselves questions to discover what we really want. We may also have to find out what our potential partners want. We don't have to have all the answers and solutions. Others can help. Why waste any more time struggling, suffering and remaining unhappy? Relief may be just a phone call, workshop, self-help book, or therapy session away.

We need to learn how to ask and how to receive the answers we get. We need to be able to truly listen and to hear what our partners say they want, not what we think they should want.

Step 8

How Can You Overcome Your Blocks And Create Joyful Intimate Sexual Relationships?

Sexual Healing

As we begin to heal the disconnection between our body, mind and spirit, we can no longer tolerate verbal abuse, tiny humiliations, control, manipulation and lack of acknowledgement from others. Whether we are in a loving relationship, an unhappy situation, or have been alone for years, as we reclaim ourselves, our desire for sexual contact is sometimes temporarily diminished. We often need to turn our focus inward, pay attention to our own self first, before going back out into the world to connect with another.

Many religions practice celibacy to help us let go of physical connection to the outside world, returning our focus back to the self, back to spirit, source, creator, God.

Our sexual organs can be powerful allies, if we let them. Listen and they will tell us all we need to know about love and our relationships. Ignore the messages, or control our bodies with our mind or our willpower, and our sexual organs will seem to betray us with their exasperating honesty.

What do we want our sexual organs to do? Perform for us? Perform for someone else? Or assist us to open our hearts, feel the love inside, and bring pleasurable sensation to ourselves and others? It's that simple. Performing brings us into our mind, away from our bodily feelings. Feelings bring us into our body. Once we connect within, it is easy to connect with others.

Your Sexual Healing

How do you want sex to be in your life?

What needs healing in your body, your mind, your emotions or your spirit?

What steps have you taken to heal your body, your mind, your emotions and your spirit?

Being Celibate For A Month, Six Months,

A Year or Longer

If you are truly serious about reawakening your sensuality and sexuality, you may choose to remain celibate for awhile, examining your life, your thoughts, and your emotions. You can use this private time to determine what you really want in a partner, a lover, a steady companion, or a lifetime mate. When you are ready, you can return to the world of sexual activity and sexual connection. After a brief hiatus, you will then be able to approach your love life with insight, wisdom and the power of knowing "I can do without it and still be okay."

What would it be like to forego sexual connection for an entire month, 30 or 31 days? What would it be like to abstain for 6 months, for one year or for longer than that? How would your lifestyle, health, energy level and emotions be affected? Some of us have already been sexually abstinent for months, years, or even decades. Some of us have never actually had any sexual experiences with others. And some of us have been seeking sexual contact for so long, with such intensity, that we often approach potential partners like a panting animal in heat. Many of us jump in and out of relationships quickly, rarely taking time between relationships to be alone, to be celibate, and to contemplate what we really want in our life.

For those of us who have rarely gone without sexual contact for even brief periods of time, **what would it be like for you to totally refrain from sexual contact for a month or longer?** Without an outlet for the accumulation of emotional and physical tensions, you might find yourself feeling agitated, nervous or depressed and lethargic. You might feel lonely, isolated, insecure about your sociability, closed off, and less interested in the world around you. You may have difficulty sleeping, your mind racing and reviewing the day, flooded with thoughts, evaluating your actions, obsessing over minor details. Without your usual and expected dose of sexual activity, you might even feel as if you are going crazy. You might find yourself obsessing about how you would compare to their current lovers. You may become overwhelmed with your fantasies, desires, longing, craving and neediness. Or, if sexual relationships have been problematic for you, you may actually find yourself sleeping better, having more energy for work, for pursuing creative projects, or for spending time with friends. You may even rediscover a forgotten interest in some hobby or other leisure activity.

You can choose to fill your time with activity, traveling, gambling, shopping, exercising, or even working. You can temporarily satisfy your sexual desires with online social networking,. You can suppress your feelings with conversation and food. Or you can suppress your feelings with mind-altering chemicals, drugs, cigarettes, or alcohol. Being celibate for awhile offers you a rare opportunity to look inside, examine your true feelings, notice the many ways you attempt to use and suppress your sexual energy. You can then focus on your dreams without the emotional complication of sexual intimacy with another person.

In a difficult relationship, sex can be the last avenue for getting close. The fear is, if you take time off from the one area of closeness between you, all sorts of bad things will happen. Actually, stopping that last link to pleasure and intimacy, you may be able to see your relationship more clearly for the first time. You may observe your partner's attributes, both favorable and unfavorable, without being swayed by your own physical desires and needs. Brief periods of refraining from sexual contact can help you to discover your own inner longing and reflect upon your own unmet needs. Then, you can begin to heal your relationship with yourself first, and then with your intimate partner/s.

Many of us can only delve so far into our own nature. To understand yourself and your relationships more fully, you have many choices. You can pursue private psychotherapy, relationship, couples and sex therapy, workshops, body therapy, and body psychotherapy, and even personal coaching.

Step 9

Making A Commitment to Your Own Sexual And Spiritual Reawakening

A Healing Journey Inward

Have you felt your heart patter lately?

Do you sense your organs smiling?

Is there a glint in your eyes and a lilt in your voice?

Does your body feel free and alive?

Do you move confidently and gracefully with strength and purpose?

If not, then maybe you are ready for a new experience.

Sexual Reawakening is the return of your body/mind system to a sensual state it once knew or may have never known. It is not measured by the frequency of sexual contact, the intensity or number of orgasms, the amount of sexual desire or the number of intimate relationships. It does not even require having a partner.

What appears to be a sexual problem in your life may not be a problem at all. The obvious symptom, unreliable erection, lack of pleasurable sensations, or inability to reach orgasm, may be used by your conscious mind as a smoke screen, a mask, a clever device to cloud and confuse the real issue. Freud and other psychotherapists have written volumes about our unconscious, neurotic and psychotic defenses. All of us are masters at hiding the truth from ourselves. But how many of us are brave enough to tackle our deception, delve into the turmoil in our minds, and strive to reach for a level of authenticity, truth and joy in our lives?

Once we journey inside to our own core, the healing process has already begun. This is what Reawakening is all about. We reconnect to those lost parts of ourselves, those parts that hold us back from good feelings, from connection, from love. Aren't we all attracted to and in awe of a person who seems self-confident and secure? Wouldn't you like to approach life, love and romance on a sure footing? Let's begin to celebrate

the joy of life and the wonder of our own precious relationships.

Your Commitment to Your Own

Sexual Reawakening

In your journal or on a clean sheet of paper, write the heading

"My Commitment To My Own Sexual Reawakening."

Close your eyes and imagine your sexual reawakening as a fête a complis, a

completed event. Imagine how you look and feel and express yourself.

Imagine the people or non-human animals, plants, or elements of nature that

are sharing your good feelings with you. Slowly open your eyes, pick up

your pen and write freely.

Do not censor your thoughts. Write whatever thoughts come to you. Read

your commitment every day. Add to it and alter it as your feelings change.

But remember, it is your commitment, your slow steady focused progress

toward your final goal that will result in transformation of your life.

Your Commitment to Your Own

Spiritual Reawakening

In your journal or on a clean sheet of paper, write the heading

"My Commitment To My Own Spiritual Reawakening."

Close your eyes and imagine your sexual reawakening as a fête a complis, a

completed event. Imagine how you look and feel and express yourself.

Imagine the people or non-human animals, plants, or elements of nature that

are sharing your good feelings with you. Slowly open your eyes, pick up

your pen and write freely.

Do not censor your thoughts. Write whatever thoughts come to you. Read

your commitment every day. Add to it and alter it as your feelings change.

But remember, it is your commitment, your slow steady focused progress

toward your final goal that will result in transformation of your life.

Step 10

Sexual And Spiritual Reawakening

At Last!

Finding a love partner in life is a blessing, a gift from God. Many of us have intense attractions toward others. Many of us have shared a romantic whirlwind of love and intimate feelings, with someone, for awhile. Then reality hits us in the face. Just those qualities that most attracted us at first are the very qualities we find irritating, agitating, boring, or even hateful, in our partners as we spend time together.

I believe we choose our partners to heal those parts of ourself that need healing. The partner who attracts us probably has certain strengths or abilities that complement the areas in which we feel we are lacking. As we get to know each other, our weaknesses, compulsive behaviors, or flaws become glaringly obvious to both of us. That's when we have the opportunity to either heal or run away.

If we stay for awhile and face our vulnerabilities and inadequacies, we have an opportunity to gain our own inner strength from our partner's outer strength. We can heal even the most deep-seated traumatic memories through loving connection with another human being. In intimate relationships we exchange energy and we feed each other with touch and love and our sexual being. In intimate relationships we have the most powerful opportunity to heal our lives.

It is also possible to solve our inner problems when we are not involved in a relationship, when we are living in an emotional hiatus between relationships. After a period of intense self-exploration, a point may come when we are ready to reconnect in a new relationship. That's when our relationships truly become a celebration of joyful connection without the fear of losing our identity.

If each of us does the inner work, self-examination and life review, the joy in our lives will be immeasurable. We will then become an inspiration to others, sharing our light and love, peace and joy with everyone who meets us.

As discussed earlier in this book, people who have gone through near death experiences, in reviewing their lives, claim they were not asked, "How much money did you make? How beautiful or sexy or intelligent were you? How many times did you have sex? How great a lover were you in bed?"

No. The only question asked was, "How did you love?" Lifetime experiences were evaluated in terms of how much love you felt and shared with others. In the end, nothing else seems to matter at all.

Sexuality is God's gift to us, teaching us how we love or don't love, through bodily experiences of exquisitely pleasurable sensations. Many of us have forgotten the true purpose of sexuality in our lives. Enhancing your senses and then gaining control over them brings you closer to your own self and to the divine. Suppressing and denying your natural senses, behaving in emotionally, physically, or sexually destructive ways, feeling uncontrolled desire, compulsively seeking thrills and promiscuous sexual adventures, usually indicates that you are disconnected from your own core. When you value non-intimate activity more than contact and intimacy, we are you are probably experiencing a split or disconnection between your mind, your body and your true spiritual self.

When you feel your connection to your own inner core, you can't help but treat all life including animals, plants, ourselves and other humans with love, respect, and compassion. You know how to love and be loved. You face each day with humility, grace and thankfulness for the gift of our very lives.

Are you ready to find your true love in yourself and with another?

Are you willing to share your own beautiful light with the world around you?

SEXUAL AND

SPIRITUAL

REAWAKENING

AT LAST!

SEXUAL AND SPIRITUAL

REAWAKENING

CHAPTER 3

SEXUAL AND SPIRITUAL

REAWAKENING ... AT LAST!

Now The Time Has Come

Now the time has come

I've spoken to my hungry heart

Unveiled its secret longing

As I carve away

The ragged edges

Of my lonely life

Senses sparkling

In the light of day

Penetrate the darkness

As its wings enfold me

Wisdom flowing outward

Cells alive, ablaze

With love

Armor dangling

By a single thread

I await the subtle signals

Of your enduring love

Transparent eyes reveal

The story of your private heart

I hear your silent words

Rumbling

In the center of my core

What are you telling me

My love?

Has your body ached

To reconnect

With something, someone

Greater than this earth

This life

This place?

Then take my hand

And let me lead you

Down the path

That we will make

Together

The time has come

My love

Let's play like children

Romping in the sun

Our hands entwined

Our hearts engulfed

Our bodies throbbing

Sensing, flowing

With delight

In love

In pleasure

Now

Sensually alive

Sexual and Spiritual

Reawakening

At Last!

Copyright © 8/14/99 Erica Goodstone, Ph.D.

Sexual And Spiritual Reawakening

Will Transform Your Life

Spiritual and Sexual Reawakening are total life-transforming events. It is not just the culmination of required rituals, disciplined practice, hard work, or specific exercises. It does not require having a partner. Spiritual and sexual reawakening is expanding and controlling all of your senses, coming face to face with your own inner being, your soul, your God essence. No place to hide. Nothing to do but let go and feel the love that has always been there. Spiritual and sexual reawakening is being reborn into life, living every day like a bright eyed, innocent child -- with awe and wonder, excitement and joy, and total aliveness.

Spiritual and Sexual Reawakening are about returning to your true self, regaining your integrity, reclaiming what is truly yours. It is about removing self-imposed boundaries and restrictions. You re-discover that love and beauty surround you - everywhere. Spiritual and sexual reawakening brings you back to nature. You open your eyes and see the forests, smell the flowers, taste the fruit, hear the wind, and touch the earth.

With all of your senses, you feel your connection to everyone and everything that exists.

Spiritual and Sexual Reawakening is a life experience. It occurs when you are in a place of total presence, aliveness and connection, to yourself, to life, and to others. It is about listening to your body, your mind, and all of your senses, observing and tempering your automatic responses.

Sexual Reawakening Is About Freedom

Sexual reawakening is about freedom - freedom to love, freedom to touch, and freedom to feel; freedom to say "yes" and freedom to say "no." It is the freedom to explore your own and your partner's bodily sensations, without shame, guilt, or embarrassment. As you gradually increase your sensual awareness, tensions in your body lessen, allowing you to tune in to your sensations and freely express your emotions. Your capacity for intimacy and creative expression naturally flourishes.

Spiritual Reawakening

Is About Freedom

Spiritual reawakening is also about freedom – freedom from the prison of automatic emotional responses, both positive and negative, freedom from your own preconceived ideas about the way life should be, freedom from your own circular mental thought patterns that keep you stuck and unable to move on, and freedom to be fully alive in every moment. As you gradually increase your spiritual awareness, your mind becomes more naturally at ease. You find yourself not holding on so much, not needing so much, not even wanting so much. Negative situations and less spiritually minded people seem to drop away from your every day experiences. Your capacity for acceptance, fulfillment, appreciation, gratitude and joy naturally flourishes.

Sexual Reawakening Is About Soul Connection

Sexual reawakening is not about keeping your eyes open and staring at your partner during sex. That's okay, but it is not essential. If it was, then all people with visual impairments would have less than adequate sexual experienceds. Even with severe visual problems, we can and many of us do, have exquisitely intimate sensual and sexual experiences.

Sexual reawakening is not about the words we communicate. If it was, then all people with speech and hearing impairments would have less than adequate sexual experiences. Even with severe speech and hearing problems, we can and many of us do, have exquisitely intimate sensual and sexual experiences.

Sexual reawakening is about soul connection. Physically challenged, mentally disturbed, and chronically ill people always retain the capacity to connect to their own soul and to their partner's soul. As long as you are conscious, as long as you are alive within your physical body, through simple touch with any or all of your senses and through intimate sexual contact, you can easily have access to your own and your partner's soul.

Spiritual Reawakening

Is About Acceptance

Spiritual reawakening is about acceptance, learning to accept and even honor each other, for all the ways we are the same and for all the ways we differ and can learn from each other. Spiritual reawakening is knowing that every person is unique with a particular family background, relationship history, lifestyle and perception of the way love is. You discover that each of us has special gifts and talents as well as inadequacies and blind spots. You learn that what is easy and natural for one person may be difficult for another.

Sexual Reawakening Is About

Exploring Your Own Unique Love Style

Sexual reawakening is uncovering and exploring your own unique love style and sexual response pattern. You learn to teach your partner/s what you want them to learn. You carefully pay attention to what your partners are teaching you about yourself, about their self, and about the world. You realize that everybody is teachable, everybody must be taught, and that YOU may have to be the example first. You understand that learning is slow and it happens step by step, day by day, experience by experience, through repetition and practice. As you continue to expand your spiritual awareness, you discover that most of us learn best when treated with compassion, kindness and patient acceptance.

Sexual reawakening is about developing the sensitivity, awareness, and patience to give and receive love with all people in your life, especially your most intimate partner/s. You discover that love is all there is. You recognize that love often brings up anything unlike itself for the purpose of release and healing. You learn to look beyond the immediate moment to unleash the unlimited potential within yourself and your chosen partner/s.

The Process Of Sexual Reawakening

Now, you are ready to begin the process of Sexual Reawakening. In the last chapter, you examined your history, your sexual desires and sexual preferences, your overall health and lifestyle, your relationship and commitment style, and what has been preventing you from creating the sexual and love relationships you have now desire. At this point, you understand what you need to do, or to stop doing, to create more fulfilling love in your life. Now you are ready to take that step into the unknown, to truly face yourself and to continue your own personal transformation that has has already begun.

Discover Every Man And Woman
In Your Partner's Eyes

Look deeply into your partner's yes and observe this precious being in front of you. If you don't currently have a partner, look in the mirror at yourown self. Stay fully present.

Discover every woman in this one woman. Discover every man in this one man.

Make love a priority. Teach each other. Love each other.

Trust that both of you can and will learn to love.

Allow love to prevail every moment of every day, every time you are together, fully clothed or fully unclothed.

Play at being lovers. Love with all your senses.

Reconnect to the joy and pleasure our sexuality was meant to be.

Once you allow this deep and loving connection to solidify, your very real partners will begin to offer the sweet ambrosia of your dreams. Every man will become the man of steel, hard as a rock, who can go all night, or at least feel as if he can -- because he won't have to perform for you, prove himself to you, try to be better for you. There'll be nothing for him to prove to anyone. Every woman will become the goddess she was born to be, regardless of her natural endowments, age or physical appearance. Watch the masks and layers of defense peel away as you peer into each other's souls. **Most of all, play and have fun!**

Your Ideal Man/Your Ideal Woman

In your journal, describe your own ideal man and your own ideal woman.

How does your current partner compare to your ideal man or woman?

If you do not currently have a partner, choose someone from the past or someone with whom you would like to become intimately involved.

How do you compare to your ideal man or woman?

How would your ideal man or woman respond to your current partner?

How would your ideal man or woman respond to you?

Reflect upon your responses.

Your Sexual Experiences

Sit quietly and take a few slow, deep, easy, and rhythmical breaths. Allow your body to relax. Begin to reminisce about a recent sexual experience. If you have not had a partner for a long time, reminisce about an experience with a previous partner or reminisce about an experience of self-stimulation.

What did you feel in your body?

What were you thinking and believing about yourself, your body, your partner, your partner's body, your responses, your partner's responses?

What did you do with your partner?

What did you say to each other?

What did you feel in your body before you started, during physical contact, and after the sexual contact ended?

Take a moment now to write your answers to the above questions in your journal or on a clean piece of paper.

Your Partner's Sexual Style

Have your partner stand and face you directly. If you do not currently have a partner or your partner is unwilling to participate in this exercise, look at a photograph of your current partner, a previous partner, or someone you would like as a partner.

As an observer, what do you notice?

Describe to your partner what you see -- physical appearance (weight, posture, shape, skin, hair, eyes), attitude and general mood (confident, insecure, worrier, angry, agitated, nervous), clothing and style.

How do you feel about your ideal partner's sexual style?

What sensations do you feel in your body?

In your journal, describe your ideal partner's sexual style and its effect upon you. Describe your ideal partner's physical appearance, attitude, approach toward you, words and sounds, behaviors and body movements, smell and taste, thoughts and feelings, style of touching and responsiveness to being touched. Describe the way your body responds.

Your Sexual Style

Stand directly facing a mirror, preferably a full length mirror in which you can see your entire body. If all you have is a small mirror, then observe your face and move the mirror around to glance at the rest of your body. Take a long slow, easy, and deep breath.

Imagine stepping outside yourself and becoming a distant observer of you, the woman or man, today, right in this moment.

As an observer, what do you notice?

Describe to yourself what you see -- physical appearance (weight, posture, shape, skin, hair, eyes), attitude and general mood (confident, insecure, worrier, angry, agitated, nervous), clothing and style.

In your journal, describe your own sexual style and its effect upon your partner. Describe your own physical appearance, attitude, approach toward your partner, words and sounds, behaviors and body movements, smell and taste, thoughts and feelings, style of touching and responsiveness to being touched. How do you feel about your own sexual style? Pay attention to your bodily reactions. Describe them now.

Your Sexuality

Our sexuality is a wonderful gift. We get to experience pleasurable and exquisite sensations. We become intimately connected with ourself and with others. But for so many of us, our sexuality is hardly pleasurable. Attempting to deny our sexual feelings, we hide behind a disinterested persona. Expressing our sexuality may cause us to feel anxious and insecure. The mere thought of sexual contact and physical intimacy may bring back painful memories and send us into a state of panic.

Sexual and sensual exploration, alone or with a loving partner, feels wonderful. Sharing yourself with another makes you feel accepted and connected. Openly sharing your deepest feelings with another helps you to know your own self, what you like and dislike, what you feel, what you want and who you are. When you allow yourself to let go and fully experience your sexual aliveness, you may have a sense that you are more than your physical body, that you are actually a powerful spiritual being.

Sexuality is the mystery of life itself. Sexuality is not only for the very sexy, the very beautiful, the sleek and slender, the very brilliant, or the very skilled man or woman. Sexuality is not only for young adults or blossoming adolescents. Even if we are hard of hearing, unable to see, barely able to talk, walking with a cane, or totally paralyzed with very little physical sensation, every one of us has sensual desires, needs and feelings.

Why then are so many of us afraid of this naturally wonderful part of life? At first glance, it may appear that our current age, our current state of health, our current partner, previous lovers, or our earliest sexual experiences are the reasons we are not enjoying our sexuality now. However, when we touch and are touched by another and when we feel sexually aroused, bodily memories fill our senses. Our bodies may recall what our minds have long forgotten: the way we were touched in our earliest moments on earth and the stimuli we received while still in our mother's womb. Reconnecting us to preverbal memories and unexpressed emotions, our sexuality, with or without a partner, becomes a direct link to the deepest part of our knowing, our inner soul.

What Is This Marvelous Thing Called Sex?

Afraid of failing, of not performing, of not appearing to be a stud or seductive vixen, many of us are turning to drugs to enhance our lagging desire and sexual arousal. Bypassing our bodily sensations, emotional needs and unique sexual response pattern, we attempt to conquer our fears and overcome our natural body responses. Here is a typical scenario of the modern quick fix style of sexual contact with our most intimate partner.

A man and woman decide to have sex one evening. Shortly after dinner, each takes a pill to enhance their own sexual arousal. Sitting and facing each other silently, they wait.... In about 45 minutes, a flush begins to cover their partner's face. That's the signal that they are both ready to have sex. They proceed to the bedroom to complete the act.

Is this what sexuality is all about? If you are a couple wanting to produce a baby, maybe taking an arousal enhancement pill can remove the fear of not being able to perform and can assist you to have sexual intercourse at the exact moment of ovulation. However, regularly relying upon a pill to become sexually intimate with a partner, is attempting to bypass and ignore your natural bodily erotic signals. Relying on a potency pill does not teach a man or woman about the nuances of what it takes to satisfy their own or their partner's sexual needs. A pill does not eliminate your sexual fears, remove your sexual inhibitions, or eradicate memories of trauma or sexual abuse.

Your Sexual Concerns

If your sexual responsivity is less than what you want it to be, it would be beneficial for you to do some self-exploration. Ask yourself the following questions:

* *What am I afraid of?*

* *Why do I need to "perform" and who am I performing for?*

* *How do I feel about my sexual partner?*

* *How do I feel about my own body, about enjoying sexual contact and orgasmic pleasure?*

* *What are my senses, my mind, and my intuition telling me about my partner, my sexuality, and my current lifestyle?*

If you attempt to bypass your anxious feelings by taking a pill, you may miss the opportunity to face your deepest fears and create lasting love and happiness in your life.

Fears and insecurities about your sexuality often prevent you from trusting your inner knowing. The answers to most of your conflicts and confusion lie in your very own body. When you pay attention to y body signals and accept the messages you receive, sexual reawakening has begun.

When you pay attention to your bodily signals, you want to communicate your needs to your partner/s. In a loving sexual relationship, there is a natural balance between attempting to please a partner and asking for what you want. But sex is not just about following instructions, like directing traffic. Many of us have been turned off to having sexual relations because our partner told us what to do, what not to do, how to feel, how not to feel. In short, someone else determined for us what our sexual behavior and emotional responses should be. Perhaps, we have been the person directing the show. In an attempt to please us, our partner's natural passion may have been suppressed. Here are some examples of words, requests and demands that may interfere with your natural sexual expression.

"Please don't. I don't want to. No, no, no…!"

"Ouch, you're hurting me!"

"Stop, I don't like when you do that!" "No, that's irritating me!"

"Touch me here. Yeah, right here. Ooh!"

"A little softer. Press here. That's right. Ahh!"

Don't move. Hold it. Stay still if you don't want me to come!"

"Is this the way you like it? Tell me what to do!"

"How was that for you? Did you have an orgasm?"

Do your most intimate sexual experiences often sound like this? Is this what sexuality is all about? Is that all there is? Do you feel as though you are always trying to please your partner or always expecting your partner to please you? Do you feel as though you or your partner can never quite get it right?

Your Senses and Your Sexuality

All of our senses are intimate. We hide our heads in shame after a wrong-doing. We do not look directly into another's eyes when we are avoiding the truth. Children hide behind mommy's skirt when they do not want to be seen. Many of us are afraid to sing or voice our own opinion in front of people. We use deodorants and colognes to avoid letting another smell us "au naturel." We wear make up to hide our blemishes and enhance our appearance.

Animals, totally accepting their own bodies and bodily functions, often delight in sniffing and licking each other's most intimate body parts – in public with no shame. Taste is one sense we usually share only with our most intimate lovers. Some of us choose not to share the intimacy of taste at all. Many of us abhor deep kissing and refuse to engage in oral-genital contact. Most of us are repelled by fluids that emanate from the nose or ears or anus, even our own. In some cultures, all the natural body fluids and sounds are seen as natural life expressions.

In some Asian cultures, belching and releasing gas through farting are encouraged as natural releases, as natural as sneezing and coughing. In these same cultures, drinking one's own urine, known as Urine Therapy, may be encouraged to increase one's natural immunity. Yogis, who have a deep connection to their own bodily functions, regularly practice numerous kriyas or cleansing techniques. To cleanse the nasal passages, they may insert a long piece of gauze into one nostril and retrieve it through the other nostril. To cleanse the throat or intestines, they often insert a long piece of gauze deep down into the throat and then slowly pull it out. Some men have practiced inserting a piece of gauze into the tip of the penis and then slowly retrieving it. More familiar to western cultures is the use of enemas and internal juice cleanses.

Your Senses and Your Sexuality

Close your eyes. Take a few slow, easy, rhythmical breaths. Allow your body to relax.

Imagine yourself being sexually intimate with your partner.

Notice what it is like for you to connect with your partner with each of your senses.

Do you enjoy the contact or do you feel uneasy, frightened, insecure, agitated, terrified, bored, or some other emotional response?

Observe how you feel and then write your responses in your journal.

* Gaze into your partner's eyes and maintain eye contact for 3 minutes

* Give and receive gentle touch, deep pressure touch, sensual touch, and sexually intimate touch

* Speak with graphic words to describe your partner's body and the way your partner's body feels to you.

* Allow natural sounds to emerge from your body and throat

* Listen to the words and sounds expressed by your partner

* Sing to your partner and listen as your partner sings to you

Breathe deeply, slowly, and in rhythmic synchronicity with your partner's breathing

Seeing, Your Partner and Sex

How does your partner look to you?

Is he or she attractive, appealing, and sexy in your eyes?

Does he or she fit your pictures of feminine or masculine beauty?

Does anything annoy, bother, disturb you or turn you off about their looks?

Hearing, Your Partner and Sex

What does your partner say to you?

How do their words feel in your body?

Do their words please, tease, titillate, excite you or turn you on?

Do their words upset, irritate, annoy, or hurt you?

How do you feel about the sound and tone of your partner's voice?

Does your partner's body or throat release sounds? How do those sounds affect you?

Tasting, Your Partner and Sex

How does your partner taste to you - sour, sweet, bitter, pungent, salty...?

Do you like the taste of your partner's skin, mouth, breath?

Do you enjoy giving oral sex to your partner?

Does your partner enjoy receiving oral sex from you?

Does your partner enjoy giving oral sex to you?

Do you enjoy giving oral stimulation to your partner's anal area?

Does your partner enjoy giving oral stimulation to your anal area?

Is there any other place you enjoy or do not enjoy tasting on your partner's body?

Is there any other place your partner enjoys or does not enjoy tasting on your body?

Smelling, Your Partner and Sex

How does your partner's smell or scent affect you?

Do you find his or her natural scent pleasing, pleasant, offensive, or unpleasant?

Do you like or dislike his or her unique scent?

Does your partner wear perfume or cologne and do you like the fragrance?

How does your natural body scent affect your partner?

Does your partner like the perfume or cologne you wear, if you do?

Touching, Your Partner and Sex

How does your partner's touch feel to you: gentle, soothing, rough, too light, ticklish, too hard, aggressive, too tentative, just right...?

How do you touch your partner?

Do you enjoy being touched by your partner?

Does your partner's touch arouse you on sexually?

Do you enjoy touching your partner?

Does your touch arouse your partner sexually?

Do you have a similar desire or need for a certain frequency and amount of touch?

Does your partner touch you only as a prelude to sex?

Do you touch your partner only as a prelude to sex?

Are you comfortable touching your partner in public?

Is your partner comfortable touching you in public?

Talking, Your Partner and Sex

What do you say to your partner during sex, during dinner, during activities, in light conversation, in heavy conversation?

Who talks more, louder, more assertively or more aggressively?

What tone of voice do you tend to use with each other?

Do either of you scream, insult, verbally abuse, humiliate and shame the other?

In what circumstances --in private, in public, with close friends, with relatives?

Can you freely say what you feel and talk about the things that matter to you?

Does your partner listen willingly and do you feel heard and understood?

Can your partner freely say what he or she feels and talk about the things that matter? Do you listen willingly and does your partner feel heard and understood?

Your Bodily Sensations

Your Partner and Sex

What sensations are you aware of feeling in your body when you are with your partner -- in non sexual situations and during intimate sexual encounters?

What body parts feel relaxed, tense, open, closed, accepted or rejected?

Your Mind, Your Partner, Love and Sex

Mind Mapping

You are about to create a map of the way your mind thinks.

Take out four clean sheets of paper or write in your journal. On four separate pages draw a large circle in the center of the page. On each circle, draw ten separate lines at the outside of the circle extending outward away from the circle.

On the first page, in the center of the circle write your own name.

Without censoring or hesitating, on each line extending outward away from the circle write a word that you associate with yourself. Whatever words come into your head, write them on one of the vertical lines pointing outward from the circle. For example, when you see your own name, you might respond with such words as: sexy, powerful, strong, inconsiderate or such words as: lazy, shy, ugly, poor, insecure. Add more lines to add more words if you need them. Now, like branches of a tree, draw additional lines extending outward from the lines you have already created, adding new words that occur to you upon observing the word already written. For example, if you have written "sexy," additional words that may occur to you are: long legs, silky hair, confidence, charming, aloof. Continue to allow the words to flow. Add additional branches as new words occur to you. You may begin with a word like ugly and branch off into poor complexion, too short, unappealing and then find words like sensitive, caring, compassionate, giving. Allow your mind to continue to make connections. Keep writing words until you feel your have exhausted your thinking process for now.

On the second page, in the center of the circle write your partner's name or, if you do not currently have a partner, write the name of a previous partner or someone you currently desire to know better. Without censoring or hesitating, on each line extending outward away from the circle write a word that you associate with yourself. Whatever words come into your head, write them on one of the vertical lines pointing outward from the circle. Add more lines to add more words if you need them. Now, like branches of a tree, draw additional lines extending outward from the lines you have already created, adding new words that occur to you upon observing the word already written. . Allow your mind to continue to make connections. Keep writing words until you feel your have exhausted your thinking process for now.

On the third page, in the center of the circle write the word "Love." Repeat the above process allowing your mind to expand upon ten different branching thoughts about love.

On a fourth page, in the center of the circle write the word "Sexuality." Repeat the above process allowing your mind to expand upon all your branching thoughts about love.

When you have finished, place all four circles in front of you and compare the words listed in each.

Notice the words you use to describe yourself, your partner, love and sex.

Reflect upon your responses.

Are there any words that you used in all four mind maps?

What have you discovered about your thoughts, ideas and beliefs about yourself, your partner, love and sexuality.

Your Spiritual Reawakening

Mind Mapping

Open to a new page in your journal. **In the center write your name**

followed by the words "Spiritual Reawakening,"

for example, "Erica's Spiritual Reawakening."

Without censoring or hesitating, on each line extending outward away from

the circle write a word that you associate with yourself as your awaken to

your own spirituality.. Whatever words come into your head, write them on

one of the vertical lines pointing outward from the circle. Add more lines to

add more words if you need them. Now, like branches of a tree, draw

additional lines extending outward from the lines you have already created,

adding new words that occur to you upon observing the word already

written. . Allow your mind to continue to make connections. Keep writing

words until you feel your have exhausted your thinking process for now.

Take a moment to compare your spiritual reawakening words to the

words you used to describe yourself, your partner, love and sexuality.

Find those words that you repeated in more than one category.

Find those words in your spiritual reawakening mind map that are missing in the other mind maps.

Reflect upon what all this might mean about what your have been focusing on, what you have been thinking you need, and what you truly value.

Letting Your Senses Speak

To Your Partner

Sit facing your partner. If you do not have a partner, face your own self in a mirror.

Actually, the only partner we ever really need is our own self and our connection to God. Now, gaze into your partner's eyes or your own eyes. Breathe slowly and deeply together with the person in front of you. Hold hands with your partner or with yourself.

Allowing Your Lips to Speak

Kiss your partner or yourself respectfully, gently, butterfly kisses on the face, eyelids, and ears.

Kiss the front, back and side of the neck, moving the hair out of the way.

Seduce your partner through your lips.

Allow your lips to speak, to sing, to tell their story, to express how much you love.

Kiss to awaken your partner's or your own soul.

Allowing Your Eyes To Speak

Kiss, caress, love and seduce your partner or yourself with your eyes.

Look with soft eyes, sensual eyes, bedroom eyes.

Feel the energy rising within you and between you, expressed through your eyes.

Define the outline of your partner's body or your own body with your eyes.

See beneath the outer appearance to the beautiful soul inside.

Breathing Your Love

Breathe deeply, slowly, and in sync with your partner's breathing.

Pant, breathe heavily, and exaggerate the motions and the sounds of your own breathing. Expand and extend your breathing.

Hold and release your breath.

Feel your breath spreading throughout your body, connecting you more fully to your partner and to your own self.

Sounding Your Love

Allow soft sounds to emerge from your throat.

Let the sounds become louder and louder.

Begin with a gentle "Ah." Say it with soft eyes and slow deep breathing.

Expand and intensify the sound of "ah."

Spread the sound of "ah" all over your partner's or your own face and body.

Make the sounds "Ay" – "Hay" – "Say"

Feel the sensation spreading through your body.

Make the sounds "Oh" - "Woh" - "Soh – "Noh."

Allow the energy to build as you say "No - o -o "

Make the sounds "Oo" and "Woo" and "Soo."

Explore your partner's and your own face and body with "ooh."

Make the sounds "Eee" - "Whee" - "See."

Observe the feelings and sensations.

Make the sounds "You -oo" - "Mou-oo " - "Wou-oo."

Feel the sensations of all the sounds opening the channels in your energy systems.

Speaking Your Sensual Love

Speak to your partner's or your own body parts, using sensual, alluring and seductive words.

I love your womanly wonderful round curves.

I love your potent powerful male body.

Say what you believe your partner's or your own body wants to hear.

Your vagina is wet and moist and open to me.

It wants to hear me talk.

Your penis is your manhood.

Let it show me how powerful you are.

Speak in a language that is not your native tongue. Exaggerate the accent.

Je t'aime mon amour.

Amore.

Let the words of passionate love open your throat. Speak from deep in your throat.

I love your strong and sexy body, my man of powerful means

I love your beautiful female body, my woman of my dreams

Practice speaking sensually to your partner as if rehearsing for a Broadway play.

Be convincing! Find the words and sounds that open your own heart and throat and loins.

Discover the words and sounds that make your partner's loins and heart long for you.

Strengthening

Your Internal Sexual Muscles

Inhale, squeeze your PC muscles, the muscles that allow you to refrain from urinating.

Exhale, release your PC muscles.

Inhale, squeeze your PC muscles, touch your partner or yourself gently.

Speak those sensual, loving words you have been practicing. Allow the words to flow from your heart.

I love your sweet sensuous smile and the soothing curves of your womanly body.

I love your masculine muscles that bulge from your hard firm frame of a man.

Exhale, release your PC muscle, continue speaking softely as you touch your partner or yourself.

Let me linger in the softness of your cheeks and sweet smelling hair.

Let me linger in your broad strong shoulders and your thick manly hair.

Kissing, Touching, Sounds and Words

Kiss your partner or yourself gently, firmly on the eyelids, cheeks, jaws, neck, throat, or behind the ears.

Caress your partner's or your own shoulders as you gently kiss the neck and chest.

Do not approach the intimate sexual body parts.

Do not blow in the ear.

Do not kiss the lips.

Do not use your tongue.

Remember - less is more!

Tease your partner's or your own body with gentle words and kisses and touches.

Touch and kiss and repeat those sensual words you have practiced for awhile.

Then be quiet, sit back, breathe together, and gaze into each other's eyes.

Moving Your Body

Put on an imaginary silk body stocking *while your partner watches or your watch yourself in the mirror.*

Brush your own hair *as you allow your head to gently move in circles.*

Bend your knees, *keeping your feet together, knees together, and hands firmly on your thighs.*

Circling your Knees

Inhale, squeeze your PC muscle and circle your knees to the right five times.

Exhale, release your PC muscle and circle your knees to the left five times.

Chopping Wood

Lift both your arms, gently arch back and imagine chopping wood.

As you bend forward, repeat the sounds as strongly as you can: Ah, Oh, Oo, Ee, Ay, Eh.

Circling Your Hips

Inhale, squeeze your PC muscle and circle your hips to the right five times.

Exhale, release your PC muscle and circle your hips to the left five times.

Move your hips in a figure 8, five times to the right and five times to the left.

Circling Your Torso

Inhale, move your torso, your upper body in a circle five times to the right.

Exhale, move your torso, your upper body in a circle five times to the left.

Rocking Your Pelvis

Inhale, move your hips forward and back five times in a pelvic rock.

Exhale, move your hips backward and forward five times in a pelvic rock.

Letting Your Partner Guide Your Body

Take turns being the mover and the person being moved. If you don't have a partner, stand in front of a mirror and imagine doing these exercises with a partner.

Put an imaginary body stocking on your partner, slowly and carefully.

Remove an imaginary sweater from your partner, caressing your partner's body.

Brush your partner's hair, sensually and lovingly.

Move your partner's knees in a circle five times to right and five times to left.

Move your partner's hips in a circle five times to right and five times to left.

Move your partner's torso in a circle, five times to right and five times to left.

Move your partner's hips in a figure 8, five times to the right and five times to the left.

Move your partner's hips five times forward and backward and five times backward and forward, in the pelvic rock.

Moving Together

Put an imaginary body stocking on both of you, slowly and carefully.

Remove an imaginary sweater from both of you, caressing your partner's body.

Brush each other's hair, sensually and lovingly.

Move your partner's hips together in a circle five times to right and five times to left.

Move your partner's torso together in a circle five times to right and five times to left.

Move your partner's hips in a figure 8, five times to the right and five times to the left.

Move your partner's hips five times forward and backward and five times backward and forward, in a pelvic rock

Female partner turn your back to the male partner, sit in his lap as both hold her knees and circle five times to the right and five times to the left.

You Are Handsome/Beautiful
Sexy And Powerful

Sit and face each other, inhale and squeeze your PC muscles, exhale, release your PC muscles and say the following words:

Woman says: *John (Say your partner's name), You are a sexy, handsome, powerful man.*

Man answers: *Yes, I am a sexy, handsome, powerful man.*

Man says: *Liz (Say your partner's name), You are a sexy, beautiful, powerful woman.*

Woman answers: *Yes, I am a sexy, beautiful, powerful woman.*

Touching and
Gazing Into Each Other's Eyes

Very, very slowly, barely moving, approach each other's faces.

If you do not have a partner, approach your own face in the mirror.

Place gentle kisses on each other's throats and necks and chest and shoulders.

With your hands, gently feel your partner's hair and head and forehead.

Now reach for your partner's lips with your lips.

Kiss the lips as if to discover every sound and every movement, every corner, every sensation, every meaning, every word.

Allow your tongue to get excited. Let your tongue begin to wonder what it would be like to explore your partner's throat.

Now gently take turns letting one person's tongue slowly, softly, gently, and fully. Explore your partner's throat and teeth and inner cheeks. Move your tongue in and out. Circle your tongue to the right, to the left, in figure 8's, and up and down.

With your tongue say,

Hello, I love you.

I'm here with you. You're safe. I'm curious and excited.

I desire you. I'm thrilled to be with you.

Taste your partner's essence with your tongue.

Gently and lightly nibble and caress your partner's lips.

With your lips and tongue and fingers say, "I love you."

Hugging Your Partner

Breathe deeply, slowly and in rhythm with your partner as you hug a full body hug.

If you do not have a partner, hug and caress your own body as fully and sensually as you possibly can.

With your partner or yourself maintain contact with as many body parts as you both can. Allow your toes and knees and thighs and pelvis touch.

Allow your hips and bellies to touch.

Let your chest and ribs and shoulders touch.

Gaze into each other's eyes and gently rub each other's cheeks and nose.

Allow your foreheads and chins to gently connect.

Press your lips together in a firm and open, gentle kiss.

Allow your hands to gently and firmly explore your partner's or your own body.

Take time to sense and feel the texture, shape and warmth of every body part you touch. Begin by caressing the neck and shoulders, arms and elbows, wrists and hands and fingers.

Move to the upper back and chest.

Allow your fingers to explore and caress the face, gently touching the eyelids, lashes, eyebrows, and cheeks.

Trace the contour of the lips.

Move your hands to the lower back and hold the belly firmly in your grasp.

Caress the hips and thighs, explore the knees and calves, ankles and feet.

Play with the toes.

Yes, it's wonderful to have a live, full-bodied partner. But, even without a partner, now you know you can always enjoy your own sensuality and sexuality. You may choose to be with another person, but you no longer need a partner to enjoy your own sensual and sexual aliveness. You can feel sensual, sexual, and happy, all alone, by yourself, at any time.

Following Your Own Senses

My toes tingle as I spread them on the floor. Outstretched arms reaching for the sky, I breathe in the morning sunlight. My yawning lips part into a beaming smile. Peering through the shutters, my waking eyes glimpse the beauty of this brand new day. Listening intently, my ears awaken to the sounds of the morning -- birds chirping, horns honking, dogs barking, people talking. The sweet fragrant scent of freshly brewing coffee boosts my morale as I quicken to ready myself. Splashing cool water on my face, I glance briefly at the image in my bathroom mirror. Stepping into the steaming shower, my voice begins to hum and sing a favorite tune. Lathering up my hands, I spread the soft aromatic soap all over my gradually awakening body. My cells filled with life, my body stretched and warmed, my pores open and receptive, I step from the shower onto the fluffy bathroom mat. Briskly drying my body with the velvety crinkly towel, I run my fingers along the soft clean fabrics soon to be embracing and enveloping my body. Dressed and ready to go, I take one final appreciative look at my own image in the full length mirror. All my morning senses satisfied, I sit down to eat a healthy balanced breakfast. My day has begun.

Sexual And Spiritual Reawakening

At Last!

Sexual Reawakening begins when you take your first breath in this world and ends with your final breath. Between those two momentous events, sensual and sexual reawakening occurs anew every moment of your life, if you pay attention and allow the sensations to build. You can choose to experience all of your senses or you can limit your sensual exposure, lessen your sensual pleasure, and prevent your sexual reawakening. We are multi-dimensional sensual and sexual beings. How sensual and sexual do you want to be? The choice is always yours, limited only by your personal beliefs, values and actions.

Yes, you can share it with a partner. Yes, you can focus on your sexual organs. And yes, all of your senses can come alive, with or without a partner, with and without sexual arousal - awakening, acknowledging, accepting, and loving your own God-given self.

By now you have discovered that it is truly a sensational world. Your senses keep you connected to the world around, your environment and the people closest to you. Your body, your mind and your imagination allow you to feel the most exquisite physical sensations and the most joyful emotions. Your senses also bring you awareness of danger and painful sensations of physical injury. Your mind can help you to withstand the pain, overcome the pain and often not even feel the pain when focused elsewhere. Your mind can also intensify the pain beyond what your senses actually cause you to feel.

Your brain is probably your most powerful sexual organ. Through your brain, you allow the flood of hormones to fill your body and arouse your senses. Your mind is even more powerful. Your mind is actually the true creator of your life. Think about it, focus on it, dwell on it, obsess about it, and you will probably bring it into being.

Nothing has ever been created without somebody first thinking about it in their mind. Do you want to create love? Then begin to focus on love in your mind, your heart, your dreams, your fantasies, your interactions, and your whole being. Do you want to create healing in your life? Then begin to focus all your attention on healing whatever you need to heal. Use your mind to imagine you are already completely well. In the future present state of mind all healing occurs, all manifestation occurs, all things are created.

What then is **Spiritual Reawakening**? You are not your body with all its moveable parts, internal organs, systems, physical sensations, pains and pleasures that you feel. You are not your calculating, intelligent brain and all its interrelated functions. You are not your emotional states.

Then who and what are you? Whether you choose to believe it or not, whether you like the idea or not, you are, always have been, and always will be, a spiritual being inhabiting a physical body. When your heart stops and your brain stops functioning, your body no longer performs its routine functions. Not one part of your body can move without your thought – even internal organs that you may never have considered having the potential to respond to your thoughts. Some of your thoughts are conscious, but much of your thinking is beyond your conscious awareness - unless you diligently practice mindful awareness.

Spiritual leaders will tell you. People who practice meditation and mindfulness will tell you. People who have had intense religious, out of body, paranormal or some type of unexplainable spiritual experiences, will all agree that we are spiritual beings. We are not just brains and bodies, interacting with others, performing our life roles, and passing from this earth. We are more than many of us choose to realize.

Knowing that you are actually a spiritual and energetic being, you realize that you are energetically connected to everyone and everything in this world and beyond. Your energy affects others. Even your thoughts, like radio waves, spread out way beyond your own brain.

Check it out. Enter a place where some negative energy is accumulating – hostility, rage, or danger. Notice how your body feels in that environment. Observe your thoughts, your energy, and your focus. Then find a place where loving, healing, positive energy is building – love, touch, kind words, compassion, and sensitivity. Notice how your body feels in that environment. Observe your thoughts, your energy, and your focus.

This book has introduced you to some concepts, beliefs and ideas that may be new to you. Maybe you have had a sense that perhaps you really are more than your body, yet you have not really explored this possibility beyond that passing thought. Maybe you are more advanced and have studied spiritual wisdom from one or many sources over a span of many years. Wherever you currently are, you can find like minded people to help you expand to a higher, more consistently fulfilling state of mind. We are all on the path to sexual and spiritual reawakening. This is a lifelong path. Enjoy the journey now.

FOOTNOTES

Chapter 1

1. Lama, Dalai, Cutler, Howard C. (1998). The Art of Happiness: A Handbook for Living. NY: Riverhead Hardcover, Penguin Books.

Chapter 2

1. Colapinto, John. (2000). As Nature Made Him: The Body Who Was Raised As A Girl. NY: Harper Collins.

2. Nevid, Jeffrey S., Rathus, Spencer A. Human Sexuality in a World of Diversity (2nd Ed.) (1995). NY: Allyn & Bacon, pp. 274-276.

CONGRATULATIONS!

You have completed Book Four in this life transforming book, *Love Me, Touch Me, Heal Me: The Path to Physical, Emotional, Sexual and Spiritual Reawakening.*

You now may realize that we are all sexual beings and that feeling your sexual aliveness reawakens you to who we are. By allowing full sexual expression into your life, you cannot help but discover your true spiritual nature. You are a spiritual being. Connecting to your spiritual nature and spiritual potential enables you to have a greater acceptance and appreciation of life. The path of discovering your spiritual connection can be difficult, painful and may reveal to us our deepest, darkest, most unloving personal attributes. Your life path is a spiritual path, the process of rediscovering your connection to all that is. No matter which direction you choose to take, all paths will eventually lead you home. Every spiritual teaching reminds us of that simple truth.

My goal in writing this book was to act as a guide and a mentor along the path of self discovery. If you resist knowing and living this truth and you decide to pursue a self-centered, ego-gratifying, and purely material way of life, you may encounter more struggle, more difficulties, and more tests than necessary. But rest assured, no matter which path you follow, you are already on your way home. My wish is for you to have a speedy, fulfilling, life affirming and joyful return home to love through physical, emotional, sexual and spiritual reawakening.

MORE TO COME!

LOVE ME ... Please

Love Me ... Please, the first book in this four part series, leads us on a path toward loving ... truly loving, from the center of our being. Love is the ultimate aphrodisiac. Love is patient, kind, unyielding, enduring and steadfast. Love overcomes all obstacles. But what most of us have called love, our human concepts and human attempts at love, with its sense of limited supply, ownership, and "what's in it for me" attitude, is filled with illusion, self-consciousness, insecurity, doubt and emotional upheaval. True love, unconditional love, a higher state of love, is limitless, boundless, and the ultimate creative power of the universe.

This book is meant for lovers, people who love, people who want to love, people who have loved, and people who want to love again. You will not find simplistic answers and easy to follow formulas for creating love. You will have to look deep into your own consciousness – your thoughts, beliefs, attitudes, memories and dreams – to find the love, the fullest love, that you can bring into your life. And you will be reminded, over and over, to bring that love back to your own self so that you can fully share your loving self with others.

Touch Me ... Please

Touch Me ... Please introduces the healing potential of simple touch, from a gentle touch on the shoulder by an acquaintance, to the warm fuzzy feeling you get when your favorite pet cuddles us to you, or the wondrously tingly sensations of your intimate lover's touch.

This beautiful Ebook is sure to delight you with powerful real-life stories about the transformative power of touch, current research, abundant exercises for self-analysis and partner sharing as well as a full explanation of the wide variety of healing body therapies and healing somatic body psychotherapies.

Heal Me ... Please

Healing happens in every moment, in every cell and organ of our body. Loving, touching, and being touched with love, we heal. When we heal, our bodies relax and our lives come into balance. In healing, we discover our own truth, face our inner spirit, and we begin to know our connection to a higher source. In *Heal Me ... Please* we examine the healing process: what we believe about healing, how we have healed our self and others, and how we can create healing in our bodies, our intimate relationships, our sexuality, and our lives.

Have any of the words or exercises in this book touched a sensitive place in your thoughts, emotions or beliefs?

Are you ready to Lose

- **Your fears?**
- **Your doubts?**

Are you ready to Create

- **Love and healing?**

It's NOT Too Late!

NOW IS THE TIME TO CREATE HEALING AND LOVE IN YOUR LIFE!

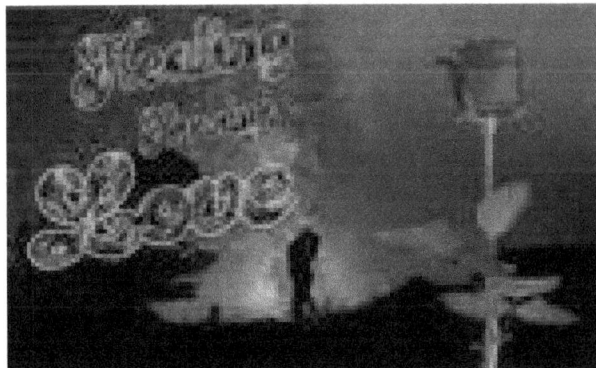

LoveNow.life/HealingThroughLoveSession

ALSO BY DR. ERICA GOODSTONE

KINDLE BOOKS

Beautiful Bare Feet: Fetish or Fantasy
Be Who You Are: The Greatest Gift of All
The Delicate Dance of Love
Your Body Believes You
It's a Sensational World
Touching Matters - The Profound Effects of Body Therapy
Let All Your Senses Speak – As You Heal
Touching Stories
Ordinary People, Ordinary Yet Extraordinary Sex
Sexual Reawakening: 10 Simple Steps
Sexual and Spiritual Reawakening – At Last!
The Science Of Being Well - Wallace D. Wattles author,
    Annotated and Illustrated by Dr. Erica Goodstone
The Science Of Getting Rich - Wallace D. Wattles author,
    Annotated and Illustrated by Dr. Erica Goodstone

Books and EBooks are available at
Amazon.com, Smashwords.com and Lulu.com

DIGITAL PROGRAMS

Love Touch Heal Video Series
Healing Through Love Audio Series
Love Lessons For Your Soul
Love Touch Heal Relationship Program

VIRTUAL SUMMITS

Men and Love Series
Women and Love Summit
Sexual Reawakening Summit
Love Me Touch Me Heal Me Summit
Healing Recovery Retreat
Miraculous Healing Master Class Summit
Science And Poetry of Love Summit
The Science of Being Well Docuseries

Programs, courses and summits available at
https://DrEricaGoodstone.com

AMAZON REVIEWS

If you have enjoyed reading this book, please consider leaving an Amazon review. The author will be most grateful because this enables her to reach more people who want to create more love in their lives.